Neurosurgical Management for the House Officer

Neurosurgical Management for the House Officer

Allan H. Friedman, M.D.

Assistant Professor
Division of Neurosurgery
Department of Surgery
Duke University Medical Center
Durham, North Carolina

Robert H. Wilkins, M.D.

Professor and Chief
Division of Neurosurgery
Department of Surgery
Duke University Medical Center
Durham, North Carolina

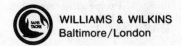

WILLIAMS & WILKINS
Baltimore/London

Editor: Carol-Lynn Brown
Design: JoAnne Janowiak
Illustration Planning: Reginald R. Stanley
Production: Carol Eckhart

Copyright ©, 1984
Williams & Wilkins
428 East Preston Street
Baltimore, MD 21202, U.S.A.

Accurate indications, adverse reactions, and dosage schedules for drugs are provided in this book, but it is possible that they may change. The reader is urged to review the package information data of the manufacturers of the medications mentioned.

Made in the United States of America

Library of Congress Cataloging in Publication Data

Friedman, Allan H.
  Neurosurgical management for the house officer.

  Includes index.
  1. Nervous system—Surgery—Outlines, syllabi, etc. 2. Nervous system—Diseases—Outlines, syllabi, etc. I. Wilkins, Robert H. II. Title. [DNLM: 1. Nervous system diseases—Diagnosis—Outlines. 2. Nervous system diseases—Therapy—Outlines. 3. Preoperative care—Outlines. WL 18 F911n]
RD593.F75 1984   617'48   84-2182
ISBN 0-683-03377-8

Composed and printed at the
Waverly Press, Inc.
Mt. Royal and Guilford Aves.
Baltimore, MD 21202, U.S.A.

Preface

This text is designed to acquaint the physician with the more common neurological disorders encountered in a neurosurgical practice. Its goal is to offer the reader a synopsis of neurosurgical problems. By presenting the text in outline form, the reader can rapidly review basic principles. It is not the intent of the authors to provide a comprehensive review of neurosurgery but rather to provide a starting point for the physician confronted with a neurosurgical problem.

While surgical technique is not discussed in this text, the medical management of patients in the perioperative period is outlined. The initial management of patients sustaining trauma to the central nervous system is also reviewed. Efforts have been made by the authors to ensure that dosage recommendations are in agreement with current practice. Because recommended dosage schedules change from time to time, it is urged that the reader check the package information for the most current recommended dose.

Allan H. Friedman, M. D.

Robert H. Wilkins, M. D.

Acknowledgments

We would like to thank Mr. Donald G. Powell for his illustrations which appear throughout this volume. Ms. Merlette B. Walker provided invaluable secretarial and editorial assistance. Mr. John F. Bolles assisted in the final compiling and editing of this edition.

We also thank the Williams & Wilkins Company for their patience and assistance.

Contents

Chapter 1

Normal Physiology

A. Cerebral Metabolism

Although the brain constitutes only 2% of the total body mass, it has a huge appetite for oxygen and glucose and utilizes a large portion of the cardiac output.

The brain uses approximately 3 ml of O_2 per 100 g of brain per minute or one-fifth of the total body oxygen consumption. If the arterial oxygen tension is lowered slowly, impaired cerebral function becomes marked below 50 mm Hg. Cerebral oxygen requirements are a function of temperature. Reducing the core body temperature from 37° to 30°C increases the amount of time that the brain can tolerate circulatory arrest from 4 to 8 minutes. Reduction of body temperature is limited by the cardiac irritability which occurs below 28°C. At 16°C, circulatory arrest can be tolerated for 30 minutes.

The brain consumes 65 mg of glucose per minute or one-quarter of the entire body's glucose consumption. Under normal conditions, the brain utilizes glucose as its only source of energy so that even moderate hypoglycemia (serum glucose < 70 mg per dl) results in brain dysfunction.

B. Cerebral Blood Flow

The normal cerebral blood flow (CBF) is about 800 ml per minute or one-fifth the total cardiac output. The average regional blood flow is 50 ml per 100 g per minute, being 65-75 ml per 100 g per minute in the gray matter and 15-20 ml per 100 g per minute in the white matter. The blood flow is a function of the cerebral perfusion pressure (CPP) and the cerebral vascular resistance (CVR).

$$CBF = CPP/CVR$$

The cerebral perfusion pressure is a function of the systemic mean arterial pressure (SAP) and the intracranial pressure (ICP).

$$CPP = SAP - ICP$$

Cerebral blood flow is compromised when the CPP falls to less than 40 mm Hg. A severe compromise in blood flow can cause physiological dysfunction (Table 1.1). The brain ordinarily can

1

maintain a constant cerebral blood flow when the mean arterial pressure is between 40 and 140 torr by modifying the intracranial vascular resistance (CVR). This is called autoregulation. The normal lower and upper limits for autoregulation are reset at somewhat higher levels in hypertensive patients.

Table 1.1.
Effect of CBF on Cerebral Function

Blood Flow	Physiological Change
16-19 cc/100 g/min	EEG change
15-16 cc/100 g/min	Loss of evoked potentials
10-12 cc/100 g/min	Cell death

Cerebral blood flow is influenced by regional need, PO_2, and PCO_2. Hypoxia results in cerebral vasodilation thus lowering the CVR, and hypocapnia causes vasoconstriction, raising the CVR.

C. Cerebrospinal Fluid Dynamics

1. CSF is principally produced by the intraventricular choroid plexus at a constant rate of about 0.35 ml per minute in adults and 0.15 ml per minute in infants. The total volume of CSF in an adult is approximately 150 ml.

2. The CSF is absorbed mainly through arachnoid villi which protrude into the venous sinuses. The rate of resorption is a function of intracranial pressure.

3. CSF can be produced and absorbed by other less clearly defined sources, e.g., across the ependymal lining of the ventricle.

4. CSF circulation: CSF flows from each lateral ventricle through its foramen of Monro to the third ventricle. The third and fourth ventricles are connected by the aqueduct of Sylvius, and the fourth ventricle communicates with the subarachnoid cisterns via the foramina of Magendie (midline) and Luschka (lateral). The CSF passes through the subarachnoid cisterns to the Pacchionian granulations, where absorption takes place (Fig. 1.1).

5. Ventricular/subarachnoid flow can be assessed by radionuclide cisternography.

THE VENTRICULAR SYSTEM

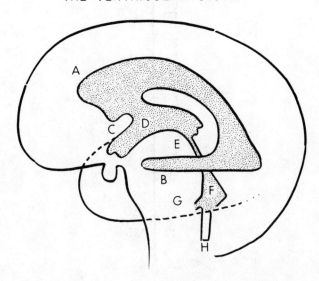

Figure 1.1. A, lateral ventricle. B, temporal horn. C, foramen of Monro. D, third ventricle. E, aqueduct of Sylvius. F, fourth ventricle. G, foramen of Luschka. H, foramen of Magendie.

D. Intracranial Volume/Pressure Relationships

A lumbar puncture measures cerebrospinal fluid pressure at one point in time. The intracranial pressure is not static. Intracranial pressure can be monitored continuously in the ventricular, subdural, or epidural space by an isovolumetric pressure transducer (Fig. 1.2).

Normal values for intracranial pressure measured at the level of the foramen of Monro with the patient recumbent:

	mm CSF	mm Hg
Adult	90 - 210	6.6 - 16
Newborn	15 - 80	1 - 6

INTRACRANIAL PRESSURE

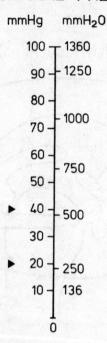

mmHg   mmH$_2$O

100 ─┬─ 1360

90 ─┼─ 1250

80 ─┤

70 ─┤ ─ 1000

60 ─┤

50 ─┤ ─ 750

► 40 ─┤ ─ 500

30 ─┤

► 20 ─┤ ─ 250

10 ─┤ ─ 136

0

Figure 1.2. Nomogram comparing intracranial pressure measurements expressed in mm Hg and mm H$_2$O. (Reprinted from Miller JD: Volume and pressure in the craniospinal axis. Clin Neurosurg 22:76-106, 1974.)

Note: If there is an intracranial mass, lumbar puncture is dangerous and can lead to uncal herniation, downward brain stem displacement, or cerebellar tonsillar herniation.

A small change in intracranial volume normally causes only a small change in the intracranial pressure (high compliance). These small changes in intracranial volume--as are normally seen with arterial pulsations, respiration, and small increases in CSF volume-- are accommodated by a compression of the veins, a distension of the meninges, and displacement of CSF into the spinal canal. After these reserves are exhausted, an increase in intracranial volume will cause a large increase in ICP (low compliance) (Fig. 1.3).

In the presence of increased intracranial pressure, a small increase in volume may cause a drastic increase in intracranial pressure.

E. Blood-Brain Barrier

The blood-brain barrier selectively regulates the passage of certain substances between the blood and the brain. It is this selectivity by which chloramphenicol readily passes into the brain but gentamicin is excluded. Tight capillary junctions, a continuous basement membrane, and glial foot processes are the anatomical basis of the barrier. Substances most likely to penetrate the barrier are those which are lipid soluble and nonionized at physiological pH. The barrier can be opened by vasodilation, by hypotonicity and hypertonicity of the blood, and by inflammation. The barrier is not fully developed at birth, as demonstrated by the vulnerability of the infant's brain to an elevated serum bilirubin level (kernicterus).

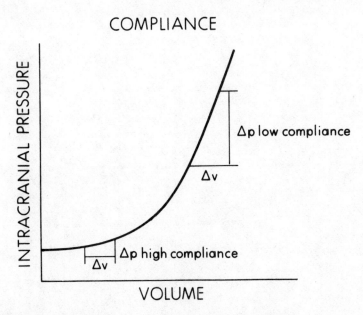

Figure 1.3. Compliance curve of intracranial contents. At elevated intracranial pressures, a small change in volume will result in a large change in pressure.

REFERENCES

Astrup J, Symon L, Branston NM, et al: Cortical evoked potentials and extracellular K^+ and H^+ at critical levels of brain ischemia. Stroke 8:51-57, 1977.

Hagerdal M, Harp J, Nilsson L, et al: The effect of induced hypothermia upon oxygen consumption in the rat brain. J Neurochem 24:311-316, 1975.

Pollay M: Review of spinal fluid physiology: production and absorption in relation to pressure. Clin Neurosurg 24:254-269, 1977.

Chapter 2

Increased Intracranial Pressure

A. Pathophysiology

Increased intracranial pressure (ICP) results from an increase in the mass within the limited confines of the cranium. Increased pressure can occur as a result of an increase in intracranial blood volume, an increase in CSF volume, cerebral edema, or a growing mass lesion (hematoma formation, etc.)

An increase in intracranial pressure unassociated with shifts of the brain produces fewer symptoms than increased ICP associated with an intracranial mass. Apparently the shift of intracranial structures produced by the mass is more important than the increased intracranial pressure in producing neurological impairment.

1. Cerebral edema is the increase in brain tissue water that results in tissue swelling. This may occur as a result of brain injury or infarction or as a reaction to a growing intracranial mass.

    a. Cytoxic edema is an intracellular collection of fluid which predominates in the gray matter and is associated with a loss of intracellular potassium. This is the type most commonly associated with a stroke.

    b. Vasogenic edema is an extracellular collection of fluid that results from an increased permeability of blood vessels. This edema accumulates primarily in the white matter and frequently remits with steroid therapy. Vasogenic edema may surround a neoplasm or a brain abscess. Computed tomographic (CT) scanning shows a sharp delineation between the cortex and white matter.

2. Vasodilation with a concomitant decrease in CVR occurs in response to the decreased cerebral blood flow seen with raised ICP. The increased intracranial blood volume due to vasodilation may further increase ICP.

3. Loss of autoregulation manifest as vascular engorgement is thought to be responsible for the increased intracranial pressure that can accompany minor head injuries in children.

4. Continuous monitoring of ICP reveals certain stereotyped
    variations superimposed upon the baseline pressure
    fluctuations. A waves are transient plateaus of increased
    intracranial pressure to greater than 50 mm Hg which last
    5-20 minutes. They are abnormal and indicate a low
    compliance within the cranial cavity. Periodic B and C waves
    occur at 1-2 per minute and 4-8 per minute frequencies,
    respectively. They occur concomitant with changes in
    respiration and blood pressure and can be seen in normal
    individuals.

B. Symptoms

1. A headache is suggestive of increased intracranial pressure
    if it is worse in the morning, wakes the patient from a sound
    sleep, is increased with exertion or the Valsalva maneuver,
    or is associated with nausea and vomiting. Headaches
    originating from a lesion in the posterior fossa tend to
    radiate to the suboccipital region.

2. Transient visual loss, especially noted with change in
    posture or the Valsalva maneuver, sometimes occurs.

3. A change in intellect or the development of lethargy does
    not seem to result from a uniform rise in intracranial
    pressure. However, these symptoms are commonly seen with
    increased pressure associated with a mass lesion.

C. Signs

1. Severe papilledema is differentiated from papillitis by the
    early loss in visual acuity seen with the latter. Both have
    essentially the same funduscopic picture. In prolonged
    papilledema, there is enlargement of the physiologic blind
    spot and concentric diminution of the visual fields. Drüsen
    bodies and retention of myelin around the nerve filaments can
    mimic papilledema on funduscopic examination.

2. Hypertension, bradycardia, and respiratory irregularities
    (Cushing's response) are sometimes present in association
    with a rapid increase in intracranial pressure or a mass
    lesion of the posterior fossa.

3. Nuchal rigidity may result from herniation of the cerebellar
    tonsils into the cervical canal.

4. Sixth cranial nerve paralysis results from a generalized
    increase in intracranial pressure and does not indicate a
    focal mass impinging on the abducens nerve.

5. Signs of brain herniation (uncal, cerebellar tonsillar, subfalcine, etc., as described in Chapter 5) do not result from an increase in pressure per se but from a pressure gradient within the intracranial cavity or between it and the cervical spinal canal.

6. The setting sun sign, a paralysis of upward gaze, is especially common in hydrocephalic infants.

7. Because the cranial sutures of children can separate, the circumference of the head will enlarge beyond the expected circumference for the child's age.

8. When the skull of a child with separated cranial sutures is percussed, it will produce a hollow sound (cracked pot sign).

. Radiographic Changes

Skull roentgenograms may demonstrate:

1. Separation of cranial sutures in children under 2 years of age.

2. Pronounced digital markings in the cranial vault.

3. Thinning of the dorsum sellae and erosion of the posterior clinoid processes in the adult skull, where the sutures are fixed.

. Treatment

1. Mechanically decreasing intracranial volume by:

    a. Decreasing the intracranial venous blood volume by elevating the head and extending the neck to facilitate venous outflow through the jugular veins.

    b. Draining CSF through a ventricular drain.

    c. Removing an intracranial mass.

2. Hyperventilating the patient to lower the PCO_2 to 25-30 mm Hg. The resultant vasoconstriction will decrease the volume of intracranial blood, thus lowering the intracranial pressure. To prevent the patient from fighting the respirator, muscle relaxation is obtained with pancuronium bromide (0.04 mg per kg, i.v.; repeat as needed). Because of its vasoconstrictive effect, hyperventilation is avoided in patients with ischemic brain disease.

3. Steroids: These agents (e.g., dexamethasone sodium phosphate 10-100 mg, i.v., then 1-4 mg, p.o. or i.v., q 6 h) are not as rapidly effective as the osmotic agents. Steroids seem to be most effective in decreasing intracranial pressure resulting from vasogenic edema that is associated with brain tumors or surgical manipulation. Steroids seem to work by stabilizing the blood-brain barrier.

4. Osmotic dehydrating agents, which cross the blood-brain barrier slowly, draw intracerebral water into the intravascular space. These agents do not decrease third space edema fluid but remove normal brain water. When the osmolarity of the brain becomes equal to the raised serum osmolarity, these agents become ineffective. The serum osmolarity of patients receiving these agents should be monitored to avoid overdehydration and renal tubular necrosis.

   a. Mannitol: Given i.v. push with a maximal effective dose of 1 g per kg q 3 h. Mannitol reduces ICP in 15 minutes and continues its effectiveness for 2-3 hours.

   b. Urea: Given i.v. 1 g per kg; works quickly but may have a rebound effect after a single dose.

   c. Glycerol: p.o. or i.v., 1 g per kg q 4-6 h is slower acting and less effective than mannitol.

5. Barbiturates: Although barbiturates seem to decrease edema formation, their precise mechanism of action remains obscure. Their initial effectiveness in reducing elevated ICP is due to vasoconstriction. The initial dose of thiopental is 3-5 mg per kg i.v. Subsequent doses are titrated to give a serum barbiturate level of 2.5-3.5 mg% (about 1-2 mg per kg q 1 h). Higher doses will precipitate systemic hypotension. EEG monitoring has been proposed as an alternative method for monitoring barbiturate administration. When an optimal dose is reached, EEG monitoring will demonstrate a burst suppression pattern cycling at 30-60 seconds. All physical parameters of brain stem function except pupillary reflexes are lost with barbiturate coma.

6. Furosemide (20 mg, i.v.) rapidly decreases intracranial pressure and CSF production. Furosemide is thought to decrease intracranial pressure by inhibiting the movement of sodium into the brain.

REFERENCES

Becker DP, Young HF, Vries JK, et al: Monitoring in patients with brain tumors. Clin Neurosurg 22:364-388, 1975.

Cottrell JE, Robustelli A, Post K, et al: Furosemide and mannitol induced changes in intracranial pressure and serum osmolarity and electrolytes. Anesthesiology 47:28-30, 1977.

Fishman RA: Brain edema. N Engl J Med 293:706-711, 1975.

Hoff JT, Marshall L: Barbiturates in neurosurgery. Clin Neurosurg 26:637-642, 1979.

Ignelzi RJ: Cerebral edema: present perspectives. Neurosurgery 4:338-342, 1979.

Lundberg N: Continuous recording and control of ventricular fluid pressure in neurosurgical practice. Acta Psychiatr Scand 36 (suppl 149):1-193, 1960.

McGraw CP: Continuous intracranial pressure monitoring: review of techniques and presentation of methods. Surg Neurol 6:149-155, 1976.

Chapter 3

Care of the Neurosurgical Patient

A. Preoperative Evaluation

1. Patients harboring a brain or spinal tumor need to be monitored closely by the neurosurgery staff in order to detect preoperative deterioration in neurological function.

2. The patient's past history should be scrutinized for surgical risk factors:

   a. Hypertensive patients have a diminished ability to maintain a constant cerebral blood flow when the systemic blood pressure is reduced.

   b. Myocardial infarction in the 3 months preceding an operation increases the risk of complications from general anesthesia to between 20 and 40%.

   c. Chronic lung disease increases the risk of operative complications.

   d. Bleeding abnormalities must be identified prior to surgery.

   e. Patients who have had prolonged bed rest have a compromised intravascular volume and are subject to hypotension when anesthetized.

   f. Certain conditions peculiar to neurosurgical patients can compromise the patient's metabolic status.

      i. Increased intracranial pressure may cause prolonged nausea and vomiting.

      ii. Steroid therapy can cause chemical diabetes mellitus and can interfere with wound healing.

      iii. Central nervous system disorders are associated with the inappropriate secretion of antidiuretic hormone. The urine osmolarity is inappropriately high for the reduced serum osmolarity. Fluid intake restriction is adequate therapy unless the

12

serum sodium is 120 mEq per liter or less, at
which point seizures may occur. If the serum
sodium is at or below 120 mEg per liter, an
intravenous infusion of hypertonic saline is
indicated.

   iv. Acromegaly may be associated with hypertension,
diabetes mellitus, and compromised cardiac
function.

   v. Cushing's syndrome may be associated with
hypertension, diabetes mellitus, and osteoporosis.

   vi. A hypothalamic tumor can cause weight loss with
loss of fat stores (diencephalic syndrome),
diabetes insipidus, or occasional hyperphagia with
marked obesity.

3. Laboratory workup should include a complete blood count,
serum electrolyte, glucose and blood urea nitrogen
determinations, coagulation studies, a urinalysis, x-ray
films of the chest, and an electrocardiogram,

4. Specific diagnostic neuroradiological, otological, and
ophthalmological studies are discussed throughout the text.
Only CT scanning of the brain will be discussed separately in
this section.

B. CT Scanning of the Brain

CT scanning of the brain is such an important and frequently
employed test in neurosurgery that special consideration will be given
to the interpretation of this examination.

A knowledge of the anatomy depicted on CT scans is an important
prerequisite for interpretation of the scans. Three representative
slices are shown as line drawings in Fig. 3.1.

Sequential Steps for the Examination of a Brain CT Scan

1. Examine the bony contours for erosion, fractures, or
hyperostosis.

2. Evaluate the ventricles for size, contour, and position. The
contour and symmetry of the ventricles may be disrupted by a
mass lesion or unilateral atrophy.

3. The pineal gland should be in the midline.

4. Abnormalities of attenuation (high or low) should be noted.
Such abnormalities usually indicate a lesion of the brain.

The gray matter normally has a higher attenuation than the white matter.

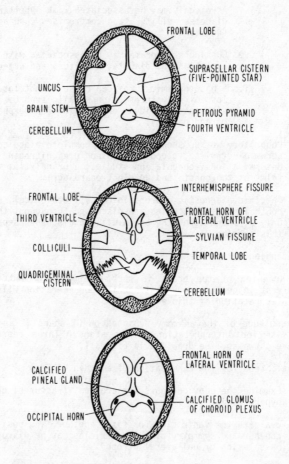

Figure 3.1. Anatomical structures shown on three successively more rostral CT scans of the brain.

5. Cortical sulci and subarachnoid cisterns are examined for evidence of enlargement (possible brain atrophy) or encroachment by an adjacent mass.

6. Lesions which disrupt the blood-brain barrier will become more prominent on the brain CT scan that is enhanced by the intravenous administration of an iodine-containing contrast agent.

   a. No enhancement: brain edema, old or very recent infarction, poorly vascularized tumor, recent hemorrhage.

   b. Dense enhancement: very vascular tumor such as a meningioma.

   c. Irregular enhancement: malignant tumor.

   d. Ring enhancement: brain abscess, primary malignant tumor, metastasis, resolving hematoma.

C. Intraoperative Problems Peculiar to Neurosurgery

1. Intraoperative venous air embolism is a possible complication whenever a patient is operated on in the sitting position. There is a potential for negative venous pressure whenever the operative site is above the level of the heart.

   Effects: Hypotension, cardiac arrhythmias, subtle pulmonary dysfunction, possible paradoxial embolism through a patent foramen ovale.

   Prophylaxis: Elevate venous pressure (positive end expiratory pressure, adequate hydration, leg wraps, or pressure suit).

   Detection: Change in sound via a precordial Doppler monitor, fall in arterial and end tidal PCO_2, an increase in pulmonary artery pressure, aspiration of air from an intra-atrial catheter.

   Treatment: Occlude venous opening (bone wax or electric cautery) and aspirate intracardiac air through right atrial catheter. If entry site cannot be detected, fill wound with saline, approximate wound edges over moist sponge, or lower head of table.

2. Intraoperative Increase in Intracranial Pressure

   During the operative procedure, the brain must be kept slack to facilitate brain retraction. A sudden increase in cerebral tension may indicate intraparenchymal or intraventricular hemorrhage.

As outlined in Chapter 2, brain relaxation can be facilitated by raising the head of the operating table, alleviating jugular vein compression, draining CSF, lowering arterial PCO_2, or administering mannitol (1 g per kg), furosemide (20 mg), or barbiturates.

3. Arterial hypotension may be induced to facilitate the dissection of an intracranial aneurysm or the resection of an arteriovenous malformation. This slackens the pressure within these delicate anomalies and lessens the chance of hemorrhage. It is important to maintain the cardiac output in the face of reduced vascular resistance in order to maintain an adequate cerebral blood flow (CBF).

Drugs for Reducing Blood Pressure	Possible Side Effects
Nitroprusside	Cyanide intoxication (tachycardia, metabolic acidosis, vascular collapse)
Trimethaphan	Histamine release (bronchospasm), tachyphylaxis
Halothane	Myocardial suppression, increased ICP
Nitroglycerin	Increased ICP

D. Postoperative Care: Cranial Operations

1. Postoperative observation is focused on changes in neurological status. It includes monitoring vital signs, level of consciousness, pupillary light reflexes, and motor capabilities. A progressive neurological deficit may be as flagrant as the onset of a hemiparesis or as subtle as a slight change in mental status.

   a. The patient should be evaluated every 15 minutes until he is awake or stable. Vital signs may then be assessed at 1-6 hour intervals, depending on the patient's condition.

   b. Blood pressure should be maintained at least at the preoperative level. An elevation in blood pressure may signal an increase in intracranial pressure, cerebral ischemia, or patient discomfort. Postoperative hypertension can frequently be treated with analgesics.

Antihypertensive therapy should be instituted cautiously, because of the risk of precipitating cerebral ischemia.

c. Changes in respiratory rhythm may indicate an enlarging intracranial mass.

d. Fever should be evaluated with physical examination, a chest x-ray film, urinalysis, and appropriate cultures.

e. Increased intracranial pressure is determined by:

i. Direct pressure monitoring which can be carried out through a ventricular CSF catheter, a subarachnoid CSF vent, or an extradural sensor.

ii. Physical signs of increased intracranial pressure and brain herniation. (See Chapter 2).

a) A full-blown Cushing response (increased blood pressure, increased pulse pressure, decreased pulse rate, irregular respiration) rarely accompanies increased intracranial pressure clinically (without brain herniation), although increased blood pressure alone is commonly seen.

b) Brain herniation: see Chapter 5.

2. Activity: Elevate the head of the bed 30°. Increase activity as tolerated. The patient may be out of bed on the second postoperative day.

3. Patient Care

a. Fluid replacement

i. Fluid overload must be avoided in an attempt to minimize cerebral edema. Intake and output charts must be maintained.

ii. 75-100 ml per hour of 5% dextrose in one-fourth normal saline + 20 mEq of KCl per liter is usually sufficient fluid replacement.

iii. Following major procedures, patients have a propensity to retain water and sodium.

iv. Normal fluid balance may be perturbed in neurosurgical patients by hypothalamic dysfunction (e.g., diabetes insipidus).

b. Nutrition: Adequate caloric intake facilitates wound
    healing and is a defense against infection. Oral intake
    may be resumed as soon as the patient is alert, except
    in those cases where swallowing may be impaired (e.g.,
    posterior fossa tumors). If oral intake is
    insufficient, most neurosurgical patients will tolerate
    tube feedings. In order to prevent aspiration,
    swallowing mechanics must be tested prior to initiating
    oral intake.

c. Seizure precautions: Although anticonvulsants are not
    routinely employed following surgery, a postoperative
    seizure should be treated quickly. If the patient has
    been on anticonvulsant medication preoperatively, this
    should be continued. Phenytoin may be given intra-
    venously, but should not be given intramuscularly. The
    absorption of phenytoin from the muscle is irregular.

d. Hygiene

    i.   Skin care: Comatose patients must be turned
         regularly, and pressure areas must be padded in
         order to avoid decubitus ulcers. Special
         mattresses and moving beds facilitate care.

    ii. Bladder care: After a craniotomy, most patients
         empty their bladder completely and only need a
         proper drainage system to keep urine off the skin.
         Patients with a concomitant spinal cord injury or
         older males with an enlarged prostate may have
         urinary retention. An indwelling bladder catheter
         may be useful while following a patient with
         diabetes insipidus.

    iii. Bowel function can be regimented with stool
         softeners and cathartics.

    iv. Pulmonary toilet includes postural drainage and
         pulmonary physiotherapy. Humidified air or oxygen
         facilitates pulmonary toilet. Comatose patients
         may require a tracheostomy for adequate pulmonary
         toilet.

4. Medications

    a. Steroids: Dexamethasone, 4 mg, p.o., or dexamethasone
        sodium phosphate, 4 mg i.v., every 6 hours or methyl-
        prednisolone sodium succinate, 40 mg, i.m. or i.v.,
        every 6 hours is used in the initial postoperative
        period to combat cerebral edema (usually for 5 days with
        an additional single repository intramuscular injection

of methylprednisolone acetate, 40 mg, or dexamethasone
acetate, 8 or 16 mg, on the fourth postoperative day).
b. Antacids (e.g., Maalox, 30 cc, p.o., every 2 hours) or
cimetidine (300 mg, p.o. or i.v., every 6 hours).

c. Analgesics: In order that the level of consciousness
can be assessed accurately, no analgesics stronger than
codeine should be given in the immediate postoperative
period.

5. Laboratory Tests

a. An immediate postoperative fall in hematocrit results
from intraoperative blood loss. A persistent decline
may result from a Cushing's (stress) ulcer.

b. The white blood count may be elevated when steroids are
administered postoperatively.

c. Arterial blood gases should be assessed to assure
adequate oxygenation and ventilation. An increased
PCO_2 level causes vasodilation and concomitant
increased intracranial pressure.

d. Serum sodium and blood urea nitrogen levels are useful
indicators of intravascular volume.

e. Electrocardiograms and x-ray films are obtained as
indicated.

E. Postoperative Care: Spinal Operations

1. The care of patients with severe spinal neurological deficits
is outlined in Chapter 10, "The Spine."

2. General postoperative care of neurologically intact patients
following a spinal operation:

a. Vital signs and examination of limb movement and
sensation every 15 minutes in the initial hours
following surgery. An epidural hematoma will lead to
progressive neurological deficit.

b. Activity: Elevate the head of the bed 30°. Increase
activity as tolerated.

c. Patient care:

i. Nutrition: Adynamic ileus may follow a lumbar or
thoracic laminectomy. Oral intake must be avoided
until this has resolved.

    ii. Intravenous fluids: 100 ml per hour of 5% dextrose in one-half normal saline until patient is taking oral nutrition.

    iii. Maintain bowel function. Do not let impaction develop.

    iv. Medications: Narcotics and analgesics may be given once the patient is awake and breathing well.

3. A patient having an extradural spinal operation without fusion is mobilized soon after the operation to avoid thrombophlebitis and respiratory complications. Large doses of analgesics are appropriate during the immediate postoperative period.

4. A patient having an extradural lumbar spinal operation with fusion is mobilized after a short period of bed rest. The patient may be mobilized in a brace or cast. Bony fusion usually requires at least 3 months.

5. Anterior cervical spine operation with fusion:

    a. Respiratory care: Because of the possibility of tracheal edema, damage to the recurrent laryngeal nerve or postoperative hematoma formation, the patient's respiratory status must be closely monitored following the operation.

    b. Dysphagia: The esophagus is usually irritated by intraoperative retraction, so the patient should initially be given a soft diet.

    c. Mobilization: The patient can be mobilized in a soft collar. Extreme neck motion should be avoided because it can result in extrusion of the bone graft. The position of the graft is assessed by x-ray films of the cervical spine in the early postoperative period and again if the patient's pain recurs.

6. Intradural spine operations without neurological deficits: Some physicians prefer to keep patients at bed rest for a few days following opening of the lumbar or thoracic dura mater in order to facilitate wound healing and reduce the possibility of a CSF leak.

REFERENCES

Horwitz NH, Rizzoli HV: Postoperative Complications of Intracranial Neurological Surgery. Baltimore, Williams & Wilkins, 1982.

Laws ER Jr, Abboud CF, Kern EB: Preoperative management of patients with pituitary microadenoma. Neurosurgery 7:566-570, 1980.

Chapter 4

Examination

A. The goal of the neurological examination is the localization of any pathological lesions within the nervous system. Some deficits can be caused by pathological lesions at any one of a number of loci in the nervous system and further investigation is necessary for accurate localization. For instance, an upper motor neuron weakness of the right leg can be caused by a lesion anywhere from the motor strip of the cerebral cortex to the pyramidal tract in the thoracic spinal cord, but when coupled with aphasia, it probably arises from a cortical lesion. If the weakness is coupled with a right third nerve palsy, it is probably secondary to a midbrain lesion, and if it is associated with a contralateral loss of pinprick sensation, it is due to a spinal cord lesion. Thus, the neurological examination of each patient is modified as abnormal findings emerge in an attempt to determine the exact location of the pathological process.

B. Examination of the patient proceeds in an orderly fashion: Higher cortical function, cranial nerves, motor function, sensation, deep tendon reflexes, and cerebellar function. Most of the examination is outlined in other sections of the book. In this chapter will be discussed miscellaneous aspects of the neurological examination.

    1. Higher Cortical Function

        a. Deficits without specific localization.

            i. Orientation (person, place, time).

           ii. General fund of knowledge.

         iii. Memory (short term memory deficit indicates bilateral lesions in the limbic system).

        b. Frontal lobe deficit:

            i. Snout, suck, palmomental, and grasp reflexes.

           ii. Change in personality.

        c. Dominant parietal lobe.

            i. Cortical sensory loss: two-point discrimination,

graphesthesia, stereognosis.

ii. Gerstmann's syndrome: impaired calculations, right-left confusion, inability to name fingers, difficulty with writing.

iii. Aphasia: see Table 4.1.

Table 4.1.
Types of Aphasia

	Broca's	Wernicke's	Conductive	Anomic
Speech	Poor	Fluent paraphasias	Fair paraphasias	Good
Comprehension	Good	Poor	Good	Good
Ability to Repeat	Poor	Poor	Poor	Poor
Naming Objects	Poor	Poor	Poor	Poor
Lesion (dominant hemisphere)	Inferior frontal lobe	Superior temporal lobe	Arcuate fasciculus	Not localized

d. Nondominant parietal lobe.

i. Dressing apraxia.

ii. Denial of deficit.

iii. Inability to copy simple diagrams (e.g., a clock).

iv. Spatial disorganization.

v. Cortical sensory loss: two-point discrimination, graphesthesia, stereognosis.

2. Cranial Nerves: see Table 4.2.

Table 4.2
Examination of Cranial Nerves

Cranial Nerve	Function	Bedside Tests and Comments
I Olfactory	Smell	Test ability to identify cigarette or coffee by odor.

Table 4.2. (cont'd)

Cranial Nerve	Function	Bedside Tests and Comments
II Ophthalmic	Vision	1. Visual acuity-Test ability to read visual acuity card or newsprint. 2. Visual fields-Check ability to count fingers or identify a small object along periphery of vision (see Fig. 4.1). 3. Examine the optic fundus.

VISUAL FIELDS

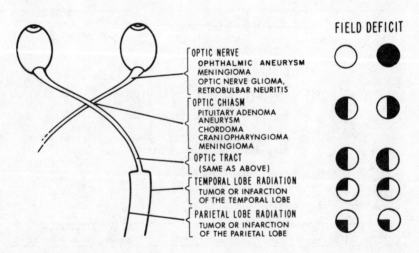

FIELD DEFICIT

OPTIC NERVE
OPHTHALMIC ANEURYSM
MENINGIOMA
OPTIC NERVE GLIOMA,
RETROBULBAR NEURITIS

OPTIC CHIASM
PITUITARY ADENOMA
ANEURYSM
CHORDOMA
CRANIOPHARYNGIOMA
MENINGIOMA

OPTIC TRACT
(SAME AS ABOVE)

TEMPORAL LOBE RADIATION
TUMOR OR INFARCTION
OF THE TEMPORAL LOBE

PARIETAL LOBE RADIATION
TUMOR OR INFARCTION
OF THE PARIETAL LOBE

Figure 4.1. Visual field deficits resulting from lesions along the optic pathway.

Table 4.2. (cont'd)

Cranial Nerve	Function	Bedside Tests and Comments
III Oculomotor	1. Eye motion 2. Pupillary constriction	1. Test extraocular motion (see Fig. 4.2). 2. Note pupillary size and reaction to light.
IV Trochlear	Eye motion (superior oblique muscle)	1. See Fig. 4.2. 2. With a third nerve palsy, the superior oblique will intort the eye on attempted downward gaze. 3. Patient with superior oblique palsy will tilt head away from the affected eye.

EXTRAOCULAR MOVEMENT

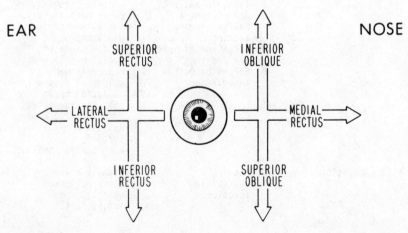

Figure 4.2.

Table 4.2. (cont'd)

Cranial Nerve	Function	Bedside Tests and Comments
V Trigeminal	1. Facial sensation 2. Muscles of mastication	1. Test sensation over forehead, cornea, maxilla, and mandible. 2. Angle of mandible not innervated by trigeminal nerve. 3. Corneal reflex blink in response to touching cornea is most sensitive and objective test of facial sensation. 4. Check muscles of mastication. On opening mouth, mandible deviates to side of V motor deficit.
VI Abducens	Eye motion (lateral rectus)	See Fig. 4.2. Abduction of eye.
VII Facial	1. Facial motion 2. Taste in anterior 2/3 of tongue 3. Salivation and tearing 4. Sensation of inner ear and tonsils 5. Stapedius muscle innervation	1. Check ability to wrinkle forehead, close eyes tightly, smile, and tense platysma. 2. Subtle signs of facial muscle weakness-enlarged palpebral fissue. 3. If facial nerve palsy is suspected, functions 2-5 can be tested by special quantitative tests.
VIII Acoustic	1. Hearing 2. Vestibular function	1. Rinne and Weber tests performed with 512 cps tuning fork.

Table 4.2. (cont'd)

Cranial Nerve	Function	Bedside Tests and Comments
		2. Observe eyes for nystagmus during extraocular movement testing or during cold water caloric response testing. 3. Obtain formal audiometry or brain stem evoked potentials if a dysfunction is suspected.
IX Glossopharyngeal	1. Sensation-posterior tongue, pharynx 2. Taste-posterior tongue 3. Salivation-parotid gland 4. Stylopharyngeal muscle innervation	Test oropharyngeal sensation and gag reflex.
X Vagus	1. Visceral and ear sensation 2. Visceral para-sympathetics 3. Pharyngeal and laryngeal muscle innervation 4. Taste (epiglottis)	Test palate elevation, gag reflex.
XI Spinal Accessory	Trapezius and sterno-cleidomastoid (SCM) innervation	1. Note trapezius on shoulder shrug. Note SCM on contralateral head turning. 2. Flaring of the scapula.
XII Hypoglossal	Innervation of muscles of tongue	Note tongue protrusion. Tongue deviates toward the side of the lesion.

3. Motor function is mediated by neurons whose axons traverse the cerebral hemispheres, brain stem, and spinal cord (upper motor neurons) and neurons whose axons traverse the peripheral nerves to end directly on muscle fibers (lower motor neurons).

   a. Mild upper motor neuron lesions will produce minor problems with coordination prior to producing enough weakness to be detected on formal examination.

   b. Upper motor neuron lesions typically produce brisk deep tendon reflexes, increased muscle tone, and an extensor plantar (Babinski) response.

   c. Lower motor neuron lesions may produce atrophy before the patient notes weakness.

   d. Rapid examination for generalized weakness.

      i. Arm

         a) Have the patient close his eyes and hold his arms outstretched with his palms facing up. Weakness will be manifested by a slow pronation and downward drift of the affected arm.

         b) With mild weakness, the patient will have difficulty performing fine rapid finger movements.

      ii. Leg weakness is best assessed by observing the patient's gait.

         a) Slight upper motor neuron weakness is manifested by external rotation of the foot and circumduction of the affected leg.

         b) The pelvis will tilt downward opposite the leg bearing weight (Trendelenburg gait) with proximal muscle weakness.

         c) Hyperadduction (scissoring) of both legs is noted with bilateral spasticity.

   e. When a peripheral nerve injury is suspected, each muscle in the affected extremity will need to be tested in order to define the pattern of the weakness (See Chapter 12, "Peripheral and Cranial Nerves").

4. Sensation.

    a. Sensory neurons are more sensitive to compression than motor neurons so that a sensory deficit may be helpful in defining subtle peripheral nerve lesions that have no concomitant motor weakness.

    b. The examination should test modalities mediated by the spinothalamic tract (pain, temperature) and modalities mediated by the posterior columns (position sensation, two point discrimination).

    c. Lesions above the thalamus will frequently spare the primary sensory modalities but may cause impaired graphesthesia (the ability to identify numbers written on the palm) or stereognosis (the ability to identify an object by touch). The patient may also demonstrate sensory extinction (if both hands are touched simultaneously, the touch on the affected hand will not be noted).

5. Deep Tendon Reflexes.

6. Cerebellar Function.

    a. Lesion in cerebellar hemisphere. Deficit ipsilateral to side of lesion. Limb difficulty with rapid alternating movements, intention tremor. Define by testing:

        i. Finger-to-nose.

        ii. Heel-to-shin.

    b. Anterior cerebellar lesion. Ataxia of gait and impairment of postural reflexes.

    c. Vermian lesion. Speech ataxia.

    d. Lesion of flocculonodular lobe. Disturbed equilibrium and nystagmus.

REFERENCES

Fisher CM: The neurologic examination of the comatose patient. _Acta Neurol Scand_ 45 (suppl 36):1-56, 1969.

Haymaker W: _Bing's Local Diagnosis in Neurological Disease_. St Louis, CV Mosby, 1969.

Patten J: _Neurological Differential Diagnosis_. London, Harold Starke, 1977.

Chapter 5

Head Trauma

A. Initial Assessment of a Seriously Injured or Comatose Patient

1. Establish an adequate airway. Clear the patient's oropharynx of debris. If oral-tracheal intubation is necessary, care should be taken not to extend the neck prior to radiological assessment of the cervical spine.

   Assess and stablize the cardiovascular system. Except in infants, intracranial bleeding cannot be extensive enough to cause shock. Persistent bleeding from a vascular scalp laceration or bleeding from a compound skull fracture with an associated dural sinus tear can be severe enough to cause shock. Occasionally a patient with a high cervical fracture and concomitant cervical-medullary junction compression will be hypotensive because of loss of sympathetic tone. However, in the usual setting, head injury does not cause shock, and another etiology should be sought.

   A history concerning loss of consciousness should be obtained. The loss of consciousness in a patient with a head injury is usually the result of cerebral concussion or contusions but sometimes stems from hypoglycemia, hypotension, inebriation, or intracranial hemorrhage which preceded the trauma. The duration of the loss of consciousness and the duration of antegrade and retrograde memory loss provide a reasonable index of the severity of the injury.

2. The initial neurological evaluation of the patient serves as a baseline for assessing future neurological improvement or deterioration. The conscious patient is given a detailed neurological examination to detect focal deficits. The examination of the unconscious patient focuses on brain stem function (Table 5.1).

Table 5.1
Assessment of Brain Stem Function

Level of Lesion	Pupils	Cold Water Caloric Response	Respiration	Movement
None	Mid-position Reactive to light	Nystagmus	Rhythmic	Purposeful
Diencephalon	Small, reactive to light	Tonic conjugate eye deviation	Yawns, pauses, Cheyne-Stokes respirations	Purposeful, decorticate
Midbrain	Mid-position, not reactive to light	Dysconjugate eye deviation	Hyperventilation	Decerebrate
Pons	Pinpoint, reactive to light	None	Apneustic breathing	Flaccid

a. Examinations of the patient's sensorium are carried out to detect progressive lethargy. The sensorium can be quantitated using the Glasgow Coma Scale (Table 5.2). A deterioration in the level of consciousness is often the first sign of a lesion which requires surgical intervention. Do not complicate or mask these changes by giving narcotics or sedatives. Besides being caused by increasing intracranial pressure (from cerebral contusions, intracranial hematomas, etc.), a decreasing level of consciousness may also be due to other factors (e.g., hypoxia, hypotension, fat emboli) that should not be overlooked.

Table 5.2.
Glasgow Coma Scale

Eye Opening	
Spontaneous	E4
To speech	3
To pain	2
Nil	1
Best Motor Response	
Obeys	M6
Localizes	5
Withdraws	4
Abnormal flexion	3
Extension response	2
Nil	1
Verbal Response	
Oriented	V5
Confused conversation	4
Inappropriate words	3
Incomprehensible sounds	2
Nil	1

Coma Score = E + M + V

b. Progressive hypertension (with widening of the pulse pressure) and bradycardia may occur as the Cushing response to increased intracranial pressure.

c. The patient's pharynx, nostrils, and auditory canals are inspected for blood diluted with CSF, a sign of a basilar skull fracture with concomitant CSF fistula. Blood behind the tympanic membrane is usually a sign of a basilar skull fracture involving the petrous portion of the temporal bone.

d. A fracture of the temporal bone extending into the mastoid may cause subperiosteal and subcutaneous hemorrhage with an ecchymosis over the mastoid process (Battle's sign).

e. Bilateral orbital ecchymoses can result from a fracture of the floor of the anterior fossa (the raccoon sign).

f. Pupillary size is indicative of the level of the lesion within the brain stem. Because of the value of the examination of the pupils in a patient with a head injury, do not give morphine, which will constrict the pupils, and do not dilate the pupils in order to see the optic fundi.

   i.   Damage of the diencephalon or pons selectively destroys sympathetic function, causing small but reactive pupils.

   ii. Damage to the tegmentum of the midbrain or third cranial nerves results in fixed, dilated pupils.

   iii. Damage involving the entire midbrain results in midposition unreactive pupils.

g. Coma from a metabolic etiology may be associated with severe signs of brain stem dysfunction, but the pupillary response to light is unimpaired. (Exceptions: Atropine or drugs such as antihistamines with an anticholinergic effect cause mydriasis; opiates cause miosis; prolonged anoxia is associated with mydriasis; glutethimide causes enlarged fixed pupils). Thus, there is a disparity between the pupillary reflexes and the other brain stem functions.

h. Vestibular-ocular reflexes are tested by lavaging the external auditory canal with iced saline (cold water calorics), after assuring the integrity of the tympanic membrane. Although ideally the patient's head is raised to 30° off the horizontal, the neck of the acutely injured patient should not be moved. Stimulation of the vestibular apparatus to test this same reflex can be accomplished by rotating the patient's head (doll's eye maneuver) but until the possibility of a cervical spine fracture is ruled out, the patient's neck should not be moved.

   i.   In the awake patient, ear lavage will cause nystagmus with the slow component toward the cooled ear.

ii. Bilateral dysfunction rostral to the third nerve
nuclei causes the fast component of the nystagmus
to be lost, and the eyes will deviate tonically
toward the side of the cold stimulus. With doll's
eye maneuver, the eyes will deviate away from the
direction of head motion and then rapidly return to
a neutral position.

iii. Midbrain lesions affecting the third nerve nucleus
or medial longitudinal fasciculus will obliterate
the adduction of the contralateral eye so that only
the ipsilateral eye moves toward the cold water
stimulus. With doll's eye maneuver, the eye
contralateral to the lesion deviates away from the
direction of the head motion, but the eye
ipsilateral to the lesion can no longer adduct.

iv. Lesions of the midpons or eighth cranial nerve
obliterate the reflex eye movements.

i. Corneal reflexes test the integrity of the fifth and
seventh nerves and their interconnection within the
brain stem.

j. Respiratory pattern is influenced by brain stem lesions.
The following respiratory patterns have localizing
value:

i. Cheyne-Stokes respirations are caused by lesions in
the basal ganglia or deep in the cerebral
hemispheres bilaterally. Lesions at this level may
cause respiratory pauses, gasps, or yawns.

ii. Hyperventilation (with normal blood oxygenation) is
characteristic of low midbrain lesions.

iii. Apneustic breathing (prolonged pauses in
inspiration) is indicative of a midpontine lesion.

iv. Nonrhythmic to and fro breathing is characteristic
of a lesion involving the medulla.

v. Loss of intercostal muscle movement with abdominal
breathing from intact diaphragm function suggests a
spinal cord injury in the lower cervical or upper
thoracic area.

k. Muscle tone, deep tendon reflexes, and motor response
are tested for asymmetry or one of the following:

i. A disparity between upper and lower extremity
movement in response to a painful stimulus

indicates a possible spinal cord lesion.

    ii. A brachial plexus injury can account for a single flaccid arm.

   iii. Loss of deep tendon reflexes in the legs or in the legs and arms suggests spinal cord injury with spinal shock.

    iv. Paratonia, a diffuse increase in muscle tone in response to passive movement, is characteristic of frontal lobe lesions.

     v. Decorticate posturing (flexion of elbows, wrists, and fingers and extension of the lower extremities spontaneously or in response to a painful stimulus) is seen with lesions in the corticospinal pathways above the midbrain.

    vi. Decerebrate posturing (extension, adduction, and hyperpronation of the upper extremities, extension of the lower extremities with the feet plantarflexed) is seen with lesions below the upper midbrain and above the vestibular nuclei.

  l. Patients with a psychiatric basis for their unresponsiveness have normal physiological nystagmus to cold water caloric testing. Their respiratory rate is normal to elevated, and their pupils react to light.

  m. Several institutions define the severity of the head lesion using the Glasgow Coma Scale (Table 5.2.). This is a rapid, reproducible method of assessing the patient's neurological function.

B. Brain Herniation (Fig. 5.1)

  l. Brain herniation can occur under the falx cerebri, through the tentorial notch, or through the foramen magnum. Downward tentorial herniation resulting from a supratentorial expanding mass can present with two different clinical syndromes. In each syndrome there appears to be a progressive loss of neurological function along the brain stem in a rostral-caudal direction. When the dysfunction is confined to the supratentorial structures, the herniation syndrome may be reversible. By the time the deficit has progressed to midbrain involvement (bilateral fixed pupils, decerebrate posturing, and dysconjugate vestibular ocular reflexes), secondary midbrain hemorrhage has probably occurred, and the deficit is usually not reversible.

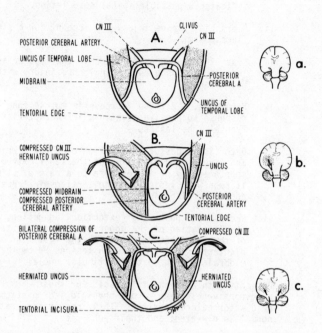

<u>Figure 5.1.</u>   Herniation syndromes.   <u>A</u>, normal anatomy at the tentorial incisura.   <u>B</u>, unilateral uncal herniation.   <u>C</u>, bilateral uncal herniation.

a. Central transtentorial herniation results from a diffuse
    increase in the supratentorial pressure or a centrally
    located supratentorial mass. The brain stem is
    displaced downward, and rostral-caudal deterioration
    proceeds as follows:

    i. The clinical signs of central herniation are
        thought to be due to a displacement of the
        midbrain and diencephalon through the tentorial
        incisura. The earliest warning of impending
        herniation is a change in mental status, i.e., a
        previously alert patient becomes confused, drowsy,
        or agitated. As the change in mental status
        progresses, the characteristic signs of forebrain
        dysfunction are seen: Cheyne-Stokes respirations,
        paratonia, small but reactive pupils. The plantar
        reflex becomes extensor (Babinski sign), and decor-

ticate posturing develops. If the patient
progresses beyond this stage, the prognosis for
complete neurological recovery is poor.

ii. If therapeutic intervention is unsuccessful,
impairment of midbrain function will occur.
Cheyne-Stokes respirations give way to
hyperventilation, and there is decerebrate
posturing. The pupils become fixed in the
midposition and the vestibular-ocular reflexes
become dysconjugate with the adducting
contralateral eye lagging behind the abducting
ipsilateral eye. Note that herniation has taken
place without a "blown" (dilated) pupil.

iii. Further progression leads to ataxic breathing, loss
of all brain stem neurological function, and
finally death.

b. Uncal herniation most often results from a laterally
placed mass pushing the uncus of the temporal lobe
medially and over the tentorial edge.

i. Dilation of the ipsilateral pupil is most often the
earliest sign of uncal herniation. Note: Although
the patient may have an altered mental status from
his initial injury or a contralateral neurological
deficit from compression of the hemisphere by the
inciting mass, uncal herniation may proceed without
a change in mental status or signs of a
supratentorial deficit.

ii. Progressive herniation results in a complete
ipsilateral third cranial nerve palsy with
impairment of extraocular motion and ptosis.
Progressive pressure on the midbrain by the uncus
at the tentorial notch is responsible for loss of
consciousness and progressive midbrain
dysfunction. Oculovestibular responses are
impaired, and ipsilateral hemiplegia may result
from compression of the opposite cerebral peduncle
against the contralateral tentorial edge.

iii. Bilateral decerebrate rigidity and hyperventilation
soon supervene. As ischemia progresses down the
brain stem, oculocephalic reflexes are completely
lost, irregular respiration occurs, and the patient
becomes completely flaccid.

      c. In unilateral transtentorial uncal herniation, the CT scan will demonstrate displacement of the midbrain contralaterally and obliteration of the interpeduncular cistern. The ipsilateral ambient cistern initially becomes enlarged but is soon filled with herniated uncus.

  2. Tonsillar herniation results from herniation of the cerebellar tonsils through the foramen magnum, most often in response to a mass lesion within the posterior fossa. Compression of the lower medulla can result in a respiratory arrest. Chronic tonsillar herniation can present as nuchal rigidity or a head tilt.

  3. Upward transtentorial herniation refers to the upward displacement of the brain stem, anterior cerebellum, and posterior third ventricle by an enlarging posterior fossa mass. Chronic herniation leads to spasticity and hydrocephalus. Acute upward herniation can lead to loss of upward gaze and a rapid loss of consciousness.

  4. Subfalcine herniation is the displacement of the cingulate gyrus under the falx cerebri. This can result in compression of the ipsilateral anterior cerebral artery. The CT scan will demonstrate enlargement of the contralateral lateral ventricle whose outflow becomes obstructed.

  5. In the evaluation of a patient with a head injury, lumbar puncture adds very little and is dangerous, because it may promote cerebral herniation.

C. Skull Fractures

  1. A linear fracture appears on plain x-ray films of the skull as a dark linear lucency with crisp, slightly jagged edges and tapering ends.

      a. Fractures must be differentiated from the complex of sutures surrounding the greater wing of the sphenoid and the mastoid. In pediatric patients, the multiple sutures and synchondroses of the occipital bone are often mistaken for fractures (Fig. 5.2).

      b. The suture line along the inner table of the skull is straighter and less jagged than the suture seen on the outer table. A superimposition of these two structures on skull films sometimes is erroneously interpreted as a linear fracture superimposed on the suture line.

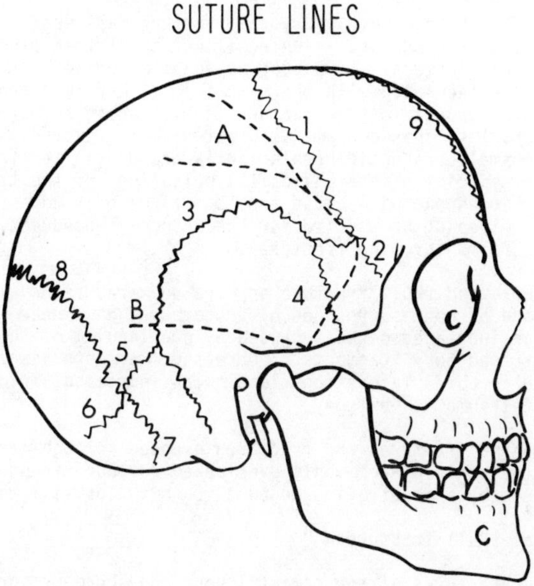

SUTURE LINES

Figure 5.2.   Pediatric skull demonstrating sutures and vascular grooves. Middle meningeal groove: A, anterior branch; B, posterior branch. Sutures: 1, coronal; 2, sphenofrontal; 3, temporosquamosal; 4, sphenosquamosal; 5, parietomastoid; 6, mendosal; 7, occipitomastoid; 8, lambdoid; 9, metopic.

Separation of the sutures, diastatic fractures, are most common in younger patients in whom an osseous closure of the sutures is still incomplete. The lambdoidal suture, which is the last to fuse, is the one most often separated.

c.   A fracture across a vascular groove may be associated with an epidural hematoma.

d.   Venous channels, unlike fractures, do not involve the full thickness of the skull, and, therefore, the channels do not appear as radiolucent on skull films. The meningeal vascular grooves follow a regular course with bifurcations and trifurcations. A familiarity with the anatomy of these grooves will prevent one from confusing them with fractures.

f. At the time of injury the fracture may gape, tearing the underlying dura. The resilient skull then closes the gap instantly, trapping adjacent material. If the scalp is lacerated with the same injury, dirt and debris can be caught in the fracture line, leading to osteomyelitis unless this contaminated material is removed. If a small arachnoid herniation is trapped in the fracture, especially in a child, the pulsations of the trapped arachnoid will cause erosion of the bony edges and widening of the fracture as seen on subsequent x-ray films (growing fracture).

2. A depressed skull fracture appears on x-ray films as an island of bone surrounded by a starburst of linear fractures or an increased density caused by overlapping of the depressed bony fragments. Depressed fragments associated with cerebral lacerations lead to an increased incidence of post-traumatic epilepsy.

3. Compound fractures are fractures exposed through lacerations in the scalp. A commonly overlooked compound fracture is one caused by a penetrating wound through the orbital roof.

4. Basal skull fractures

   a. Fractures of the parietal bone and squamous portion of the temporal bone may extend into the petrous portion of the temporal bone as a <u>longitudinal fracture.</u> These fractures are associated with tears of the tympanic membrane, disruption of the auditory ossicles, and, in some cases, facial nerve injury. The facial weakness associated with longitudinal fractures, especially when it is delayed in onset, usually recovers spontaneously.

   b. Fractures through the occipital squamosa may continue across the foramen magnum and traverse the petrous pyramid. These fractures may destroy the cochlear-vestibular apparatus and facial nerve, leading to permanent hearing loss and facial palsy. CSF is present behind the intact tympanic membrane.

5. In infants the so called "derby hat" or "ping-pong ball" fracture represents a greenstick fracture of the skull. Although the skull is indented, no fracture line is seen on x-ray.

D. CSF Fistulas

   1. Fractures of the petrous pyramid may be associated with the
      leakage of CSF out of ear through the torn tympanic membrane
      or, if this membrane is intact, leakage into the pharynx
      through the eustachian canal.

   2. CSF can escape through fractures of the walls of the para-
      nasal sinuses associated with dural tears. This occurs most
      frequently with fractures involving the ethmoid sinuses,
      which are tightly adherent to the dura mater and olfactory
      bulb.

   3. Meningitis may result from an undetected fistula.

   4. The diagnosis of a CSF communication must be suspected when
      plain x-ray films demonstrate intracranial air or an
      air-fluid level within the sphenoid sinus. CSF rhinorrhea is
      differentiated from nasal mucus by its higher glucose
      content.

   5. If the fracture responsible for the CSF rhinorrhea cannot be
      visualized on skull films and by tomography, the fistula may
      be localized by identifying the path of a radioactive tracer
      instilled into the CSF or by visualizing the route of escape
      of similarly injected metrizamide by means of computed
      tomography.

E. Injuries to the Brain

   1. The combination of skull fractures and brain contusions seen
      after a direct head injury is best described by the forces
      involved at the time of the injury. Although the mechanism
      of injury does not affect treatment, a knowledge of these
      mechanisms will provide insight into how injuries evolve.

      a. Abrupt deceleration of a moving head is characterized by
         a relatively minor injury of the brain at the site of
         impact (coup lesion) and an extensive contusion of the
         brain opposite the point of impact (contrecoup injury).
         Contusions are most likely along the undersurface of the
         frontal lobes, the tips of the temporal lobes, and along
         the falx, wherever the brain abuts an irregular surface.
         The skull may remain intact. This type of injury
         results when a moving head strikes a fixed windshield.

      b. Abrupt acceleration of an unsupported head occurs when
         the head is struck by a moving object. The skull
         accelerates against the brain causing an extensive coup
         injury of the brain. The remainder of the brain may
         remain uninjured.

c. If a well supported skull is struck by a moving object, there is little movement of the skull or brain. Most of the force is absorbed by the skull, which will fracture. Damage to the underlying brain results from direct perforation or laceration by the skull fragments.

Taking these three mechanisms into account, it is easy to understand why some of the most severe cerebral contusions occur without concomitant skull fracture and why patients who present with spectacular skull fractures are often awake with only minor neurological dysfunction.

2. Cerebral concussion is the term used to describe transient impairment of neurological function such as alteration of consciousness, disturbance of vision, etc. caused by a mechanical force. Repeated concussion, as suffered by boxers, can produce a permanent deterioration in intellect. Recent studies indicate that many patients with moderate concussions are left with long lasting mental impairments.

3. A cerebral contusion is a pathological lesion of the brain characterized by hemorrhage, necrosis, or tissue tears. Contusions can be demonstrated on CT scan as subcortical wedge-shaped areas of low density which may be speckled with blood. The term diffuse axonal injury is used to describe the widespread damage to axons in the white matter of brain which can occur with angular acceleration.

F. Intracranial Hematomas

1. An epidural hematoma is a collection of blood between the bone and dura.

a. Etiology: Epidural hematomas are usually arterial in origin, especially resulting from a laceration of the middle meningeal artery associated with a fracture in the squamous portion of the temporal bone. The tenacious adhesion of the dura to the skull in the very young and in the very old protects these age groups from epidural hematomas. Occasionally epidural hematomas stem from tears in the superior sagittal or transverse sinus. These venous hematomas accumulate slowly and may not become symptomatic for several days.

b. Symptoms: The epidural hematoma produces focal symptoms by local cortical compression but more frequently acts as an expanding mass precipitating transtentorial herniation. The classic story is triphasic with a mild head injury leading to a transient loss of consciousness followed by a so-called "lucid interval" where the patient is relatively symptom free. Consciousness is once again lost when the expanding epidural hematoma

leads to uncal herniation. This "lucid interval" may
not occur if the initial head injury is responsible for
a more prolonged loss of consciousness. In fact the
classic triad is only seen in 10% of patients with
epidural hematomas.

c. Diagnosis: Most epidural hematomas are associated with
    a skull fracture. A skull fracture seen crossing a
    vascular groove on plain skull films is cause for
    concern. The acute epidural hematoma presents on CT
    scan as a lens-shaped lesion of high density adjacent
    to the skull and sharply demarcated by the dura, which
    is firmly attached to the bone at the edges of the
    hematoma. Although cerebral dehydrating agents may
    temporarily alleviate the effects of the growing
    hematoma, in some cases there is no time for
    radiological studies, and exploratory burr holes are
    made for diagnosis and decompression.

2. Subdural hematomas are blood collections which occur in the
    potential space between the dura and the arachnoid.

    a. Etiology: Unlike epidural hematomas, subdural hematomas
        are usually venous in origin. Because of the lack of
        adhesions, blood in the subdural space quickly spreads
        out over the convexity of the brain. If the initial
        blood collection is small enough to go unnoticed, the
        clot may lyse and become enveloped by a membrane of
        fibrous tissue and friable capillaries. Thus the clot
        evolves into a chronic subdural hematoma. These friable
        capillaries, especially in the outer membrane, may
        continue to leak blood into the subdural collection,
        enlarging the mass. Subdural hematomas may occasionally
        be of arterial origin, in which case the patient's
        clinical presentation is identical to that of an
        epidural hematoma.

    b. Symptoms:

        i.   Acute subdural hematomas present as an evolving
             intracranial mass. When a small subdural hematoma
             accompanies severe brain contusion, the hematoma
             contributes minimally to the patient's poor
             neurological condition.

        ii. Chronic subdural hematomas present with an altered
             mental status, a focal neurological deficit,
             headache, seizures, or a mass effect. An often
             encountered presentation is that of a waxing and
             waning mental status in an elderly patient or an
             alcoholic. The traumatic episode causing the
             subdural hematoma is often trivial and forgotten.

      iii. In children, chronic subdural hematomas may result in frontal bossing and enlargement of the middle fossae. Chronic subdural hematoma is a cause of head enlargement in infancy. Other signs of child abuse must be sought.

  c. Diagnosis of Subdural Hematoma

      i. Clinical examination: a progressive neurological deficit, usually with an alteration in the mental status or the level of consciousness.

      ii. Skull roentgenograms.

         a) Less than 50% have an associated fracture.

         b) A calcified pineal gland may be shifted away from the midline.

      iii. CT scan.

         a) Subdural hematomas may obliterate the underlying cerebral sulci.

         b) The mass effect may shift the ventricles, but 15-20% of subdural hematomas are bilateral, in which case the ventricles may be compressed but not shifted in relation to the midline.

         c) Acute subdural hematomas have an increased density.

         d) Chronic subdural hematomas (more than 2 weeks in duration) are of low density. The membranes may enhance following the intravenous injection of iodinated contrast material.

         e) Subdural hematomas of an intermediate age or those occurring in patients with a low hematocrit may be of the same density as the brain parenchyma. These can only be detected by the mass effect they cause.

G. Treatment of Scalp, Skull, and Brain Injuries

  1. <u>Scalp lacerations</u> can almost always be repaired primarily after thorough cleansing; careful visual and sterile digital examination for foreign material, depressed skull fractures, etc.; and debridement of frankly necrotic tissue. However, if there is much tissue loss, the scalp edges may not come together, even with wide undermining, and a scalp flap or

skin graft of some type may be necessary. Hemostasis of the vascular scalp can be obtained by compressing the lacerated scalp edge against the skull. Reapproximation of the muscular aponeurosis (galea on the underside of the scalp) is necessary for a strong closure, but buried sutures should not be used in a contaminated wound where they might serve as foci for infection.

2. Linear fractures need no immediate surgical intervention.

3. Depressed fractures displaced more than 1 cm in depth should be explored unless the depression is over a dural sinus. Removal of bone fragments tamponading a torn dural sinus can be associated with massive blood loss. Bone fragments are elevated and cleansed, necrotic brain is debrided, the dura is closed, and any scalp laceration is repaired.

4. Compound fractures demand surgical debridement in an orderly fashion, with debridement of contused brain, closure of the dura, removal or cleansing of loose bony fragments, and closure of the scalp.

5. In areas of excessive bone loss, an acrylic cranioplasty is performed for cosmetic purposes and to protect the brain. In children under 5 years of age, the dura may spontaneously regenerate the lost cranium.

6. Traumatic cerebrospinal fluid fistulas usually stop spontaneously. Patients with rhinorrhea or otorrhea are monitored for signs of meningitis. Persistent CSF rhinorrhea can be treated with head elevation and continuous spinal CSF drainage, unless a tension pneumocephalus is created by the entry of air into the head. Surgical repair is indicated if the leak shows no tendency toward stopping after 7-14 days or if the patient suffers repeated bouts of meningitis. Repeated bouts of meningitis can also occur as a result of an occult dural tear without overt leakage of CSF.

7. Management of closed head injury (head injury with intact skull and scalp).

    a. Patients with no significant headache, lethargy, or focal neurological deficit can be released into the custody of a reliable relative or friend who has been instructed as to the warning signs of neurological deterioration.

    b. Patients suffering moderate head injury manifest by lethargy or severe persistent headache should be admitted to the hospital for observation.

    c. Patients with severe head injury or persistent neurological abnormalities need the following:

i. Attention to maintenance of an adequate airway and ventilation, and restoration of normal blood pressure. Pulmonary function may be compromised by aspiration pneumonia, contused lung, shock lung, pulmonary embolism, fat embolism, or (rarely) neurogenic pulmonary edema.

ii. Periodic neurological examinations.

iii. Evaluation for visceral or major limb trauma.

iv. Appropriate laboratory studies to evaluate the patient's metabolic status (complete blood count, arterial blood gases, EKG, serum glucose and calcium).

v. Plain skull x-ray films with special attention given to skull fractures, air-fluid levels in the paranasal sinuses, the presence of intracranial air, and the midline position of the calcified pineal gland.

vi. A lateral film of the cervical spine prior to moving the patient to detect unstable spine fractures. All seven cervical vertebrae must be visualized. Skeletal traction should be used for the initial reduction and immobilization of unstable cervical fractures.

vii. Chest and abdominal x-ray films.

viii. Computed tomography when available. This is the single most helpful study in the rapid evaluation of the patient with a closed head injury.

ix. Prophylaxis against tetanus if indicated.

x. Intracranial pressure monitoring with aggressive treatment of elevated intracranial pressure. This has been demonstrated to decrease the mortality of patients sustaining closed head injuries.

xi. Possible surgical intervention for an intracranial hematoma or for an acute extracranial injury (e.g., ruptured spleen).

d. Comatose patients need special care.

i. Fluid replacement: Avoid fluid overload by using 75 ml per hour of 5% dextrose in one-fourth normal saline + 20 mEq KC per liter. If the syndrome of inappropriate secretion of antidiuretic hormone

(SIADH) develops, further fluid restriction may be necessary.

   ii. SIADH is diagnosed when the urine osmolarity remains elevated in the face of a low serum osmolarity. This laboratory picture can also be seen when the patient has been given a low molecular weight agent (e.g., ε-aminocaproic acid, mannitol, etc.).

   iii. Maintain caloric intake via tube feedings.

   iv. Avoid urinary retention, cutaneous pressure ulcers, fecal impaction, and serum electrolyte imbalance (see Chapter 3).

   v. Begin antacids to avoid peptic ulcers.

  e. Sedatives and analgesics may interfere with serial neurological evaluations. Codeine, which causes minimal central depression, is the most potent agent which should be used.

  f. Evoked potentials have been demonstrated to be useful in predicting the ultimate neurological outcome in patients with closed head injuries. The prognosis of patients with normal or mildly abnormal evoked potentials is good.

8. Treatment of Subdural and Epidural Hematomas:

  a. Most of the time an extracerebral hematoma is on the side of an enlarged pupil (partial third cranial nerve palsy). If an emergency decompression must be done prior to diagnostic studies, the side of the enlarged pupil must be explored first.

  b. An acute or subacute clot is stiff in consistency and cannot be adequately drained through a burr hole. It must be removed through a large craniectomy or a craniotomy.

  c. Chronic liquified hematomas may be washed out and drained through a small opening in the skull, such as a burr hole.

  d. If a chronic subdural hematoma recurs, treatment may necessitate a craniotomy and partial removal of the enveloping membranes, or the shunting of the subdural fluid into the pleural or peritoneal space.

H. Sequelae of Closed Head Injuries

1. Early post-traumatic epilepsy occurs during the first week
    following a closed head injury in 5% of hospitalized
    patients. A delayed seizure disorder will develop as a
    neurological sequela of head injury in 5% of patients.
    Early seizures (occurring in the first week following
    injury), prolonged post-traumatic amnesia, an intracranial
    hematoma, a depressed skull fracture, or a penetrating
    injury all predispose the patient to late seizures.

2. The postconcussional syndrome consists of headaches, hyper-
    acusis and dizziness, and some reduction in memory and concen-
    tration. This syndrome is frequently seen after mild head
    injuries. Formal psychological and vestibular testing has
    demonstrated that cognitive and vestibular impairment may
    persist for months following even mild head injuries.

I. Pediatric Head Injuries

1. The prognosis in pediatric closed head injuries is much
    better than in adult closed head injuries. Even children who
    are totally flaccid and without brain stem reflexes at the
    time of admission may make a satisfactory recovery.

2. Pediatric patients who have loss of consciousness with a head
    injury are less likely to have an intracranial blood collec-
    tion and more likely to have diffuse cerebral swelling than
    are adults. Such swelling, which probably represents loss of
    normal cerebral vascular autoregulation and reactivity
    initially, and cerebral edema later, may occur rapidly in a
    child with a closed head injury and may be fatal if not
    treated quickly and effectively.

J. Gunshot Wounds

1. Cerebral destruction is influenced more by the velocity of
    the missle than by its mass.

2. High velocity bullets, as used in military conflicts, cause a
    momentary marked increase in intracranial pressure leading to
    orbital roof fractures and transient uncal herniation.

3. In civilian low-velocity bullet injuries, delayed
    deterioration may result from intracranial hematoma or
    abscess formation.

4. Treatment consists of debridement of the wound and removal of
    intracranial debris. All indriven bone fragments should be
    removed. The dura is then closed, as is the overlying scalp.

5. Copper-encased bullets are more likely to cause adverse changes in the surrounding brain (including cerebral necrosis with bullet migration, and abscess formation) than are hardened lead bullets.

6. Retained contaminated bone fragments may result in delayed intracerebral abscesses. Retained metal fragments can also harbor bacteria but are less likely to cause abscess formation.

7. Post-traumatic seizures are common.

K. Vascular Complications Associated with Closed Head Injuries

1. A dissecting aneurysm of the internal carotid artery should be considered when a patient with a closed head injury presents with a focal neurological deficit but has a normal CT scan.

2. A traumatic carotid-cavernous sinus fistula may become apparent soon after injury or may be delayed in onset for days or weeks. The patient may note a bruit, conjunctival edema and chemosis, impaired extraocular motion, and loss of visual acuity.

3. Traumatic intracranial aneurysms are a rare manifestation of trauma.

REFERENCES

Becker DP, Miller JD, Young HF, et al: Diagnosis and treatment of head injury in adults. In Youmans JR: Neurological Surgery, ed 2, Philadelphia, WB Saunders, 1982, vol. 4, pp 1938-2083.

Cartlidge NEF, Shaw DA: Head Injuries. London, WB Saunders, 1981.

Greenberg RP, Newlon PG, Hyatt MS, et al: Prognostic implications of early multimodality evoked potentials in severely head injured patients. A prospective study. J Neurosurg 55:227-236, 1981.

Jennett B, and Teasdale G: Management of Head Injuries, Philadelphia, FA Davis, pp 239-244, 1981.

Marshall LF: Nonoperative treatment of head injuries. Clin Neurosurg 29:312-325, 1982.

Miller JD, Sweet RC, Narayan R, et al: Early insults to the injured brain. JAMA 240:439-442, 1978.

Plum F, Posner JB: Diagnosis of Stupor and Coma, ed. 3, Philadelphia, FA Davis, 1980.

Rose J, Valtonen S, Jennett B: Avoidable factors contributing to death after head injury. Br Med J 2:615-618, 1977.

Seelig MD, Becker DP, Miller JD, et al: Traumatic acute subdural hematoma: major mortality reduction in comatose patients treated within four hours. N Engl J Med 304:1511-1517, 1981.

Chapter 6

Brain Tumors

Primary brain tumors arise from the neuronal elements, glial elements, and connective tissue.

A. Glial Tumors

1. Gliomas arise from the normal glial elements of the nervous system. They are:

   a. Astrocytes are the interstitial cells which play an active part in the structure and metabolic activity of the central nervous system (CNS).

   b. Oligodendrocytes are the cells responsible for producing and maintaining the myelin covering of the axons within the CNS.

   c. Ependymal cells line the ventricles and central canal of the spinal cord.

   d. Microglia are the scavengers of the CNS, analogous to the body's reticuloendothelial cells.

   e. Choroid epithelium lines the choroid plexus of the ventricles.

2. Astrocytomas of the cerebrum are slow growing, infiltrating tumors with poorly defined borders. This tumor represents the benign end of a spectrum of astrocytic tumors. Anaplastic astrocytoma and glioblastoma are the more malignant forms of astrocytic tumor. The peak incidence of astrocytomas is during the fourth decade of life.

   a. Histology: Hypercellular; unordered nuclei in a sea of eosinophilic astrocytic processes which are sometimes interrupted by microcysts.

   b. Clinical presentation: Seizures, headaches, increased intracranial pressure, or focal neurological deficit indicative of the area of the brain affected.

    c. CT scan: Low density with irregular margins crossing the gray-white matter junction; occasional calcification; minimal irregular enhancement.

    d. Treatment: Surgical resection. Radiation therapy is of value in partially resected lesions.

    e. Prognosis: Four year average survival, but patients less than 30 years old have a 5-year survival of 80%.

3. <u>Anaplastic astrocytomas</u> are more malignant than astrocytomas. They have a peak incidence in slightly older patients than do astrocytomas.

    a. Histology: Increased nuclear polymorphism and frequency of mitosis; occasional necrosis.

    b. Clinical presentation: Same as astrocytoma.

    c. CT scan: More mass effect and more enhancement than astrocytoma; interspersion of high density with low density on unenhanced scan.

    d. Treatment: Surgical resection and radiation.

    e. Prognosis: Two-year average survival.

4. <u>Glioblastoma multiforme</u> is a highly malignant glial tumor occurring most frequently in the frontal and temporal lobes. It is the most common glioma and occurs most frequently in the fifth and sixth decade of life, with a slight male predominance. This tumor can metastasize through the subarachnoid space.

    a. Histology: Hypercellular; polymorphic nuclei; palisading of cells around areas of necrosis; areas of hemorrhage and of endothelial proliferation.

    b. Clinical presentation: Increased intracranial pressure, seizures, focal neurological deficit indicative of the location of the tumor. Because the tumor frequently crosses the corpus callosum to involve both frontal lobes, personality changes are not unusual.

    c. CT scan: Mixed high- and low-density areas on unenhanced scan with significant mass effect; dense, irregular, sometimes ring-shaped enhancement.

    d. Treatment: Surgical resection, radiation, chemotherapy (1, 3-bis (2-Chloroethyl)-1-nitrosourea (BCNU) most effective).

e. Prognosis: Average survival less than 1 year.

5. Ependymomas of the cerebrum are fleshy tumors with well defined borders. They occur at the same frequency in all age groups, although ependymomas account for a much higher percentage of the cerebral malignancies seen in children and adolescents. They may metastasize through the subarachnoid space.

a. Histology: Unpatterned hypercellular tumor; the cells have eosinophilic cytoplasmic processes which may surround blood vessels (pseudorosettes); occasional regions of columnar cells radiating around a clear lumen (rosettes).

b. Clinical presentation: Headaches in younger patients and seizures in older ones. Focal findings indicate the location of the lesion.

c. CT scan: Similar to the pattern of malignant astrocytomas.

d. Treatment: Surgical resection and radiation.

e. Prognosis: Average postoperative survival of 5 years - some long-term survivors.

6. Oligodendrogliomas are slowly growing gliomas with calcifications that can often be seen on plain skull films. These tumors occur more frequently in the anterior cerebrum and have a peak incidence at 40 years of age.

a. Histology: The cells have a characteristic perinuclear halo. Fine capillaries and calcium deposits are frequently present.

b. Clinical presentation: Seizures are by far the most common presentation. Occasionally signs of a focal neurological deficit or increased intracranial pressure are seen.

c. CT scan: High-density calcified areas interspersed with low-density glioma.

d. Treatment: Surgical resection.

e. Prognosis: Average survival 10 years after the onset of symptoms (there are many long term survivors).

7. Hypothalamic gliomas are low-grade tumors which occur most frequently in children. Patients present with signs of hypothalamic dysfunction (profound emaciation, hyperkinesia,

hypoglycemia, hypotension, or precocious puberty) or a visual deficit. The tumors are of low density on CT scan. The location of these tumors precludes total excision in most cases, and most are treated with radiation therapy.

8. Optic gliomas are tumors of the optic nerve or chiasm. They occur prior to age 15 in 85% of patients, and 15% occur in conjunction with von Recklinghausen's disease. Patients present with progressive amblyopia. Tumors within the orbit produce proptosis. Skull films demonstrate an enlarged optic foramen if the tumor extends into the foramen. The CT scan demonstrates enlargement of the optic nerve or chiasm. Treatment of an optic nerve glioma is often surgical excision, although the operation may be delayed until the eye is completely blind. Lesions of the optic chiasm are treated more conservatively.

9. Gliomatosis cerebri is a condition in which malignant astrocytes are found diffusely in large areas of the central nervous system.

10. Gangliogliomas are mixed tumors containing both glial and neuronal elements.

11. Microgliomas, which present during the fifth and sixth decades, are rare tumors except among recipients of renal transplants and other immunosuppressed patients. These tumors most frequently occur in the cerebrum and present with raised intracranial pressure or symptoms referable to the location of the tumor.

12. Choroid plexus papillomas usually occur in the ventricles (especially in the region of the trigone of the lateral ventricle during the first decade of life and the fourth ventricle in adulthood).

   Clinical presentation: Hydrocephalus.

   CT scan: High density, speckled intraventricular lesion with marked contrast enhancement.

B. Meningiomas

   Meningiomas account for about 15% of intracranial neoplasms and have a predilection for adult females. These tumors are usually attached to the dura and are clearly demarcated from the brain. The tumor contains variable amounts of calcification and receives the majority of its blood supply from dural vessels. Intracranial meningiomas occur most often in a parasagittal location, over the convexity of the cerebrum, on the sphenoid wing, along the olfactory groove, above the sella turcica, or in the posterior fossa.

1. Clinical presentation:

   a. Convexity and parasagittal tumors present with headache, seizures, urinary incontinence, or a focal neurological deficit reflecting the site of the tumor. The parasagittal frontal location predisposes to gait disturbance and urinary incontinence.

   b. Medially placed sphenoid wing and suprasellar meningiomas present with gradual unilateral or bilateral visual loss. Encroachment into the orbit results in proptosis.

   c. Anosmia, the most frequent early sign of an olfactory groove meningioma, is often overlooked. These lesions come to clinical attention because of raised intracranial pressure, encroachment on the optic nerves, mental deterioration, or seizures.

   d. Posterior fossa meningiomas present with signs of cranial nerve dysfunction or obstructive hydrocephalus.

   e. Meningiomas occurring at the foramen magnum present with signs of spinal cord or brain stem compression.

   f. The rare intraventricular meningiomas present with increased intracranial pressure.

2. Pathology: Meningiomas are irregularly nodular tumors which indent the brain. They may invade the cranium, stimulating dense reactive bone proliferation. Meningiomas display several histological patterns and are classified as meningotheliomatous, transitional, fibrous, and angioblastic.

3. Radiology: Meningiomas frequently can be detected on plain x-ray films of the skull because of hyperostosis, tumor calcification, or increased vascularity of the bone adjacent to the tumor. The uncontrasted CT scan frequently demonstrates a sharply demarcated lesion which is most often hyperdense but may be iso- or hypodense. The tumor usually lies in juxtaposition to bone or to the falx and contains variable amounts of calcium. Homogeneous enhancement is seen after intravenous contrast enhancement.

   Angiography is performed to delineate the tumor's vascular supply and to determine if adjacent dural sinuses are patent or infiltrated with tumor.

4. Treatment: Surgical excision, the treatment of choice, cannot always be accomplished because of the relationship of the tumor to the dural sinuses (especially the superior

sagittal sinus) or the growth of the tumor into the bone at the base of the skull.

C. Metastatic Tumors

1. Approximately 15-20% of cancer patients will have intra-cranial metastases at the time of autopsy.

    a. Pathology: Lung, breast, kidney, and skin (malignant melanoma) are the most frequent sources of intracranial metastases. Cerebral metastases usually begin at the junction of the gray and white matter.

    b. Clinical presentation: Increased intracranial pressure (not only from direct tumor growth; metastases to the cerebellum may cause obstructive hydrocephalus), seizures, focal neurological deficit. Spontaneous hemorrhage into the tumor may occur with malignant melanoma, choriocarcinoma, or renal cell carcinoma, resulting in an abrupt onset or worsening of symptoms.

    c. CT scan: Circumscribed, often enhancing mass surrounded by cerebral edema. The rim of the tumor may enhance more than its necrotic center.

    d. Treatment: Surgical extirpation if solitary and accessible; otherwise steroid medication and radiation therapy. The role of chemotherapy remains undefined.

    e. Prognosis: 40% of patients with "single" intracranial metastases and limited systemic disease live 1 year after treatment.

    f. Meningeal carcinomatosis, the diffuse spread of a metastatic tumor through the subarachnoid spaces, is most frequently due to leukemia, lymphoma, or breast carcinoma. It presents as headache, changes in mental status, cranial nerve palsies, or radiculopathies (pain or nerve dysfunction). One may need to examine the spinal fluid several times before tumor cells are detected. Treatment consists of intrathecal methotrexate and radiation therapy.

D. Other Conditions

1. Colloid cysts are pedunculated round masses occurring in the anterior third ventricle. They present with intermittent headaches, obstructive hydrocephalus (dementia, incontinence, gait disturbance), or short-term memory loss. On CT scan, the cysts usually appear as high-density round lesions.

2. Von Recklinghausen's disease and tuberous sclerosis may present with CNS tumors.

    a. Von Recklinghausen's disease.
       i. Skin: Café au lait spots, axillary freckles, subcutaneous neurofibromas, and schwannomas.

       ii. Peripheral nervous system: Plexiform neurofibromas, schwannomas, malignant schwannomas.

       iii. Central nervous system: Schwannomas of cranial and spinal nerves, meningiomas, ependymomas, optic gliomas, gliomas.

       iv. Other abnormalities: Kyphoscoliosis, skeletal abnormalities, unusual meningoceles, benign gastrointestinal tract tumors, endocrine tumors.

    b. Tuberous sclerosis is a rare congenital disorder in which sclerotic benign lesions are found in the cerebral cortex and calcified benign tumors are found lining the ventricles. Occasionally astrocytomas are present. The CT scan demonstrates multiple periventricular high-density areas. Clinical manifestations include:

       i. Cutaneous lesions: Adenoma sebaceum, shagreen patches, subungal fibromas, and depigmented areas.

       ii. Mental retardation.

       iii. Seizures.

       iv. Tumors of the heart, kidney, and retina.

E. Posterior Fossa Tumors

Approximately 60% of the brain tumors of childhood are located in the posterior fossa. These include astrocytomas of the cerebellum and brain stem, medulloblastomas, ependymomas of the fourth ventricle, and, less commonly, choroid plexus papillomas and dermoid and epidermoid tumors.

Of primary adult brain tumors, about 25% are infratentorial. Acoustic neuromas, meningiomas, epidermoid cysts, and, less frequently, choroid plexus papillomas and glomus jugulare tumors occur in the cerebellopontine angle. Hemangioblastomas, metastatic carcinomas, and medulloblastomas occur within the cerebellar parenchyma. Ependymomas, choroid plexus papillomas, and, rarely, meningiomas appear in the fourth ventricle.

1. Tumors of the posterior fossa can present with a medley of symptoms and signs, depending on the structures most affected.

   a. Headache: May be generalized or occasionally limited to the suboccipital region.

   b. Cerebellar dysfunction:

      i. Ipsilateral ataxia and incoordination from lesions involving the lateral neocerebellum.

      ii. Unsteadiness of gait and truncal ataxia from lesions involving the vermis and anterior cerebellum.

      iii. Loss of equilibrium and nystagmus from bilateral floccular-nodular lesions such as occur with medulloblastoma.

   c. Hydrocephalus is common because of the obstruction of CSF flow. In children, this results in separation of suture lines and an expanding head circumference. In adults, symptoms and signs of hydrocephalus - such as apraxic gait, urinary incontinence, or changes in intellect - or of increased intracranial pressure - such as headache, nausea, and papilledema - may be present.

   d. Torticollis, head tilt, and neck stiffness may develop secondary to displacement of a cerebellar tonsil into the cervical canal. A head tilt may also occur in association with a trochlear nerve palsy.

   e. Cranial nerve palsies occur with intramedullary lesions of the brain stem and with tumors involving the cranial nerves directly. The sensory nerves are more sensitive to compression than are the motor nerves. Sixth nerve palsies can result from increased intracranial pressure without direct nerve involvement.

2. Medulloblastomas are malignant tumors of the vermis and fourth ventricle encountered most frequently during the first decade of life. There is a male predominance. A second peak in the incidence of medulloblastoma occurs in young adults, when the tumor more commonly presents in the lateral cerebellar hemisphere.

   a. Pathology: Soft gray tumor; highly cellular with scanty cytoplasm, hyperchromic nuclei, and occasional rosettes.

    b. Clinical presentation: Obstructive hydrocephalus with concomitant nausea and vomiting; nystagmus and gait dysequilibrium are seen with fourth ventricle tumors; hemispheric tumors cause ipsilateral incoordination; rarely, subarachnoid metastasis into the spinal canal causes the first symptoms.

    c. CT scan: Demonstrates enlargement of the fourth ventricle by a nonhomogeneously enhancing tumor; concomitant hydrocephalus.

    d. Treatment: Consists of extensive surgical resection and radiation therapy to the entire neuraxis. Recurrent tumor may be responsive to chemotherapeutic agents.

    e. Prognosis: Only one-third of patients survive longer than 10 years. Survival is enhanced by gross total removal of the tumor followed by radiation therapy.

3. Ependymomas of the posterior fossa originate from the floor of the fourth ventricle, fill the ventricle, and then occasionally extend out into the cerebellopontine angle and cisterna magna. This tumor is most common during childhood but a small number occur during the fifth and sixth decades of life.

    a. Clinical presentation: Obstructive hydrocephalus, dysequilibrium of gait, rarely involvement of lower cranial nerves or spinal metastases.

    b. CT scan: Multilobulated, irregularly enhancing tumor in fourth ventricle.

    c. Therapy: The tumor should be resected surgically, but total extirpation is rarely possible. Postoperative radiation therapy is mandatory.

    d. Prognosis: Mean survival is 2.5 years.

4. Brain stem gliomas occur most frequently between the ages of 5 and 8 years.

    a. Pathology: Widening of the pons by the intraparenchymal astrocytoma; progression to glioblastoma is not uncommon by the time of autopsy.

    b. Clinical presentation: This tumor presents with palsies of fifth through ninth cranial nerves, gait unsteadiness, and long tract signs. Sixth and seventh cranial nerve palsies are the most frequent presentations. Hydrocephalus is a rare and late finding.

      c. CT scan: Demonstrates posterior displacement of the fourth ventricle, obliteration of the prepontine cistern, and abnormal densities within the brain stem.

      d. Therapy: Radiation therapy.

      e. Prognosis: Mean survival 2-3 years.

5. Cerebellar astrocytomas have a peak incidence between the ages of 5 and 9 years. They are usually confined to the cerebellum but occasionally extend down a peduncle into the brain stem. The tumors remain well circumscribed and frequently are associated with a cyst.

      a. Pathology: The tumor is composed of loosely packed astrocytes which aggregate around blood vessels to provide a bimodal appearance.

      b. Clinical presentation: Cerebellar dysfunction and eventual obstructive hydrocephalus.

      c. CT scan: Reveals displacement of the fourth ventricle, a nodule of tumor which may or may not enhance, and in about one-half the cases a large, low-density, laterally placed cyst.

      d. Treatment: This tumor can be completely resected in 80% of cases; complete resection usually results in cure. Even partial resection has a reasonable prognosis.

6. Choroid plexus papillomas are encountered in the fourth ventricle of adults and in the trigone of the lateral ventricle in children.

      a. Clinical presentation: The tumor presents with symptoms associated with hydrocephalus.

      b. Treatment: This soft tumor is amenable to surgical excision. Care must be taken to remove the portions of the tumor that pass through the foramen of Luschka into the cerebellopontine angle on each side.

7. Hemangioblastomas are the most common primary intra-axial tumors found in the posterior fossa in adults.

      a. Pathology: Multiple tumors may arise in the posterior fossa. The tumors are pink, although sometimes yellow, and are frequently associated with a large cyst. They are composed of thin-walled vessels and lipid-laden cells.

b. Clinical presentation: The tumor presents with signs of
    cerebellar dysfunction. Sometimes hemangioblastomas
    occur as a manifestation of Lindau's syndrome:
    hemangioblastomas of the cerebellum, retina (von
    Hippel's disease), brain stem, spinal cord; congenital
    cysts of the kidney, adrenal, pancreas, lung, liver,
    epididymis; adenomata of the adrenal and kidney; and
    renal cell carcinoma. About 10% of patients with a
    cerebellar hemangioblastoma have polycythemia.

c. Treatment: Surgical excision of the tumor nodule is
    usually possible but may be quite hazardous when the
    tumor extends into the brain stem.

F. Tumors of the Cerebellopontine Angle

The cerebellopontine angle contains the fifth, seventh, and
eighth cranial nerves, petrosal vein, and anterior inferior cerebellar
artery. The medial wall is formed by the cerebellum, pons, and sixth
cranial nerve. Caudal to the angle is the jugular foramen and the
ninth through eleventh cranial nerves. Tumors originating in this
region present with cranial nerve palsies.

1. Tumor types:

a. Acoustic neuromas, arising from the vestibular portion
    of the eighth nerve, are the most common tumors found in
    this region. This histologically benign tumor presents
    with tinnitus, unsteadiness, and a slowly progressive
    hearing loss. The patient first notes difficulty
    deciphering speech through the affected ear. As the
    tumor enlarges, the corneal reflex becomes diminished on
    the affected side, indicating trigeminal nerve compres-
    sion. Because of the resiliency of the facial nerve,
    facial weakness is a rare sign of acoustic neuroma.
    Further tumor enlargement leads to brain stem and
    cerebellar compression manifested by vertigo, rotary
    nystagmus, and gait ataxia. Hydrocephalus occurs when
    the brain stem is severely distorted.

b. Meningiomas of the cerebellopontine angle may present
    with the same signs as an acoustic neuroma, but the
    signs evolve in a different sequence. There may be
    marked involvement of the fifth, seventh, or ninth
    through twelfth cranial nerves.

c. Epidermoid cysts (cholesteatomas) also occur in the
    cerebellopontine angle. Any of these three tumors
    (acoustic neuroma, meningioma, epidermoid cyst) can
    cause trigeminal neuralgia.

2. Diagnostic tests:

   a. Plain films of the skull and petrous tomograms
      demonstrate definite erosion of the internal auditory
      canal in about 80% of patients with acoustic neuroma and
      may demonstrate calcification or hyperostosis in
      association with a meningioma.

   b. The CT scan will demonstrate most neuromas larger than
      1 cm in diameter as an enhancing lesion.

   c. Stapedius reflex test is abnormal in about 85% of cases
      of acoustic neuroma.

   d. Brain stem evoked potentials are superior to audiometric
      testing in diagnosing acoustic tumors.

   e. Positive or negative contrast cisternography, combined
      with computed tomography, is the most sensitive test for
      demonstrating small acoustic neuromas.

G. Pituitary Tumors

   1. Presentation

      a. Endocrine presentation:

         i. Cushing's syndrome is predominantly a condition of
            females manifested as truncal obesity,
            hypertension, and diabetes mellitus. Patients also
            have accelerated atherosclerosis, skin striae,
            ecchymoses, wasting of the extremities, osteopenia,
            and emotional lability. The syndrome may result
            from an adrenocorticotropic hormone
            (ACTH)-secreting pituitary tumor (Cushing's
            disease) or extrasellar tumor, an adrenal tumor, or
            the iatrogenic administration of steroids. The
            diagnosis of Cushing's disease is made by demon-
            strating a loss of the normal pituitary-adrenal
            axis suppression by exogenous steroid adminis-
            tration.

         ii. Acromegaly (gigantism in children) results from an
             excess of growth hormone. Adults demonstrate an
             excessive periosteal new bone formation (manifested
             by a large mandible and a protuberant forehead),
             soft tissue thickening, and joint pain. More
             advanced cases have aberrant glucose metabolism,
             cardiovascular disease with hypertension, peri-
             pheral nerve entrapments, and myopathy. Children
             grow exceptionally tall. The diagnosis is made by
             demonstrating an elevated basal serum growth

hormone level which is not suppressed by hyper-
glycemia.

iii. Hyperprolactinemia, a disorder almost exclusively
of young females, presents as amenorrhea and
galactorrhea. The diagnosis is confirmed by an
elevated serum prolactin level. Elevation of serum
prolactin levels to less than 125 ng per ml can be
caused by diseases other than pituitary tumors.

iv. Nelson's syndrome, hyperpigmentation and a
pituitary tumor, occurs in about 10% of cases where
bilateral adrenalectomy was performed for treatment
of Cushing's syndrome. The disinhibited ACTH-
secreting tumor often behaves in a malignant
fashion. The hyperpigmentation is diffuse but is
most pronounced over joints and in recently formed
scars.

v. Hypopituitarism can result from compression of the
pituitary by an enlarging, nonsecreting tumor.
Short stature reflects diminished growth hormone
levels in children. Hypogonadism is the first sign
of hypopituitarism in adults.

b. Mass lesion:

i. Compression of the optic chiasm by a pituitary
tumor most often causes a bitemporal hemianopsia,
but other visual field deficits can occur depending
on the exact relationship of the tumor to the optic
nerves, tracts, and chiasm.

ii. Lateral extension of the tumor can lead to facial
pain and numbness or abnormalities in extraocular
motion. Invasion into the temporal fossa can
incite seizures, and superior extension can result
in hypothalamic syndromes or profound personality
changes.

c. Pituitary apoplexy, an acute massive hemorrhage into a
pituitary tumor, may mimic subarachnoid hemorrhage or
suppurative meningitis. Presentations include sudden
headache, altered level of consciousness, stiff neck,
impaired vision, and abnormal extraocular motion.

2. Diagnosis of Pituitary Tumor

a. Radioimmunoassays for pituitary trophic hormones
demonstrate elevated levels of hormone. Elevated
hormonal levels which are produced by pituitary tumors

may sometimes be suppressed by normal physiological mechanisms.

b. The sella turcica should measure no more than 17 mm from the tuberculum to the dorsum sellae on a plain lateral x-ray film of the skull. Polytomography can demonstrate irregularities in the floor of the sella turcica not seen on plain films. These irregularities are seen in the presence of all but the smallest tumors.

c. CT scanning, especially in the coronal plane, is useful in demonstrating suprasellar tumor extension. With the development of better scanners, this modality is becoming more useful in demonstrating intrasellar lesions as well.

d. Angiography is used to distinguish an intrasellar or suprasellar aneurysm from a nonsecreting tumor. This modality is also used to define the position of the carotid arteries prior to trans-sphenoidal surgery.

3. Treatment

a. Surgical resection is the treatment of choice for most lesions. The trans-sphenoidal approach can be employed for all intrasellar tumors and for adenomas extending directly above the sella turcica. Complications of this approach include cerebrospinal fluid fistula with a risk of meningitis, diabetes insipidus, cranial nerve palsies, optic nerve damage, and vascular injury. Larger eccentrically growing tumors are approached through a frontal craniotomy. This approach has most of the same risks associated with the trans-sphenoidal operation plus the risks inherent to any craniotomy.

Radiation therapy, 4,000-5,000 rads in 5-6 weeks, is most frequently used as an adjuvant after surgical resection in the treatment of larger tumors. Because radiation frequently causes an initial swelling of the tumor, radiating a large undecompressed pituitary tumor may be associated with further loss of vision.

Medical therapy: The use of bromocriptine, the dopaminergic agonist, in treatment of prolactin-secreting pituitary microadenomas is gaining popularity. This therapy is frequently used in young females with amenorrhea, galactorrhea, and elevated serum prolactin levels. It is used as adjuvant therapy in tumors which cannot be totally resected. Cyproheptadine is occasionally used to suppress ACTH secretion in patients with Cushing's disease.

4. Special Perioperative Problems

   a. Acromegalics may have accelerated atherosclerosis, hypertension, cardiac myopathy, and diabetes mellitus which should be assessed prior to an operation.

   b. Patients with Cushing's syndrome may also have hypertension and diabetes mellitus.

   c. Compression of the normal pituitary gland by a tumor may abolish the normal elevation of glucocorticosteroids that occurs in response to stress. This capacity is especially precarious following resection of the tumor. Patients should be given glucocorticosteroids in the immediate preoperative period (200 mg cortisone acetate b.i.d. for 48 hours). Following surgical stress, patients are given maintenance doses of cortisone acetate (25 mg q a.m. and 12.5 mg q p.m.) until the endocrine reserve is evaluated and confirmed to be normal. (Daily cortisone acetate will need to be increased at times of stress.) Failure to replace lost steroid function may result in Addisonian crisis (fever, nausea, prostration, circulatory collapse, diminished serum sodium level, hypoglycemia). Patients may also need replacement of thyroxine (levothyroxine sodium 0.1-0.2 mg daily), testosterone (testosterone enanthate 200 mg, i.m., bimonthly), or estrogen (Premarin O.S., 1.2 mg daily).

   d. Diabetes insipidus (DI) may be transient or permanent. No therapy should be instituted until it is certain that the patient has DI and not just a postoperative diuresis.

      i. Other causes of polyuria.

         a) Osmotic diuresis (e.g., mannitol, ε-aminocaproic acid, diabetes mellitus).

         b) Fluid overload (e.g., intraoperative fluids, polydypsia).

         c) Renal causes (diuretics, low potassium level, high serum calcium level, renal disease).

      ii. Therapy should not be instituted unless:

         a) Serum sodium is higher than 148 mEq per liter.

         b) Serum osmolarity is elevated and higher than urine osmolarity.

iii. Treatment

    a) Partial DI

        1) Chlorpropamide - up to 500 mg per day.

        2) Clofibrate - 500 mg, p.o., q.i.d.

    b) Transient DI

        Aqueous pitressin 5 units, i.m., q 6 h or when
        urine output is greater than 200 ml per hour
        for 2 hours.

    c) Permanent DI

        1) Pitressin tannate in oil 5 units, i.m.,
            two to three times per week.

        2) DDAVP - 15-25 mg intranasally b.i.d.

5. Differential Diagnosis

    a. The empty sella syndrome denotes an enlarged sella
        turcica filled with cerebrospinal fluid. This is
        usually due to the sellar extension of an arachnoid
        pouch. The arachnoid pouch may compress the pituitary,
        causing minor endocrine abnormalities. The condition is
        benign but must be distinguished from an intrasellar
        tumor.

    b. Craniopharyngiomas most frequently occur above the sella
        turcica. Although they are one of the most common
        supratentorial tumors of childhood, 50% of these tumors
        appear in adults.

        i.   Clinical presentation: Visual abnormalities, such
             as bitemporal hemianopsia due to compression of the
             visual system at or adjacent to the chiasm, partial
             hypopituitarism (most commonly, reduced
             gonadotrophins), small stature, obstructive hydro-
             cephalus (headaches, vomiting, papilledema).
             Diabetes insipidus is usually a late sign.

        ii. Pathology: Grossly irregular lobulated mass with
             calcifications and cysts which contain brown fluid
             and cholesterol crystals.

        iii. Radiology: Plain x-ray films demonstrate supra-
             sellar calcifications in 90% of children and 50% of
             adults with craniopharyngioma. CT scans demon-

strate a solid or cystic suprasellar tumor with calcifications and with some enhancement of the solid portions of the tumor.

iv. Treatment: Surgical excision is ordinarily attempted, but because of the tenacious bond between the tumor and the neural structures, bits of tumor are usually left behind. Postoperative radiation therapy is beneficial.

c. Germinomas occurring in the suprasellar region frequently present first with diabetes insipidus.

d. Meningiomas can also present as suprasellar masses.

H. Pineal Region Tumors

Pineal tumors come to clinical attention by compression of adjacent structures.

1. Presentations include:

a. Ocular manifestations of midbrain compression, such as Parinaud's syndrome (paralysis of conjugate upgaze with varying degrees of paralysis of ocular convergence and pupillary constriction), convergence spasms, upper lid retraction, anisocoria, impaired pupillary light reflex with retention of reaction with convergence, and retraction nystagmus.

b. Compression of the aqueduct of Sylvius resulting in hydrocephalus with concomitant nausea, vomiting, papilledema, and lethargy.

c. Cerebellar compression causing truncal ataxia.

d. Precocious puberty.

2. Pathology: Five classes of tumors arise in the pineal region:

a. Germ cell tumors frequently occur in the pineal region. Typical teratomas (containing representative tissue from all three germinal layers), dermoid tumors, and epidermoid tumors are benign lesions. Germinomas, which occur predominantly in males under 30 years of age, are the most common tumors found in this region. These lesions are malignant and can both invade surrounding structures and metastasize through the CSF pathways. Other germ cell tumors, such as embryonal carcinoma or choriocarcinoma, may also occur in this region.

b. Pinealomas and pineoblastomas are rare tumors which originate from pineal parenchymal cells. Pineoblastomas are the more malignant variety.

c. Tumors of glial origin may arise from the quadrigeminal plate.

d. Arachnoid cysts, meningiomas, and medulloblastomas occur in this location.

e. Vein of Galen aneurysms result from the drainage of an arteriovenous malformation into an expanded vein of Galen. This lesion may present as congestive heart failure in infancy. In older children it may present as a pineal region mass with concomitant hydrocephalus.

3. Diagnosis: Plain skull films may reveal signs of increased intracranial pressure or abnormal pineal calcification. Calcification of the pineal in patients under 10 years of age or a calcified mass in the pineal region larger than 10 mm in diameter in any patient is suspicious for a tumor. The CT scan reveals a posterior third ventricular mass and obstructive hydrocephalus. Small lesions cause only an identation into the posterior third ventricle on the CT scan. Arteriography reveals displacement of the posterior choroidal arteries and the precentral cerebellar vein. Certain tumor markers, such as α-fetoprotein and human chorionic gonadotropin, may be found in the spinal fluid of patients with a germinoma. A postoperative rise in the CSF levels of these substances may be the harbinger of tumor recurrence.

4. Treatment: Ventricular shunting alleviates the symptoms of obstructive hydrocephalus. These tumors may be exposed through a supracerebellar infratentorial or a medial occipital supratentorial approach, so that the 25% of pineal region tumors that are resistant to radiation therapy may be identified and resected and so that the radiosensitive malignant tumors such as germinomas may be reduced in size surgically before radiotherapy is given (to lessen the tumor burden for such treatment). Germinomas have also proved responsive to chemotherapeutic regimens such as cisplatin, bleomycin, and vinblastine.

Table 6.1.
Normal Values for Pituitary Hormones

Hormone	Normal Hormone Level	
Growth Hormone(GH)	Unstimulated	1-5 ng/ml 3 serum
	Stimulated (L-dopa, hypoglycemia)	5 ng/ml rise in serum GH

Table 6.1. (cont'd)

Hormone	Normal Hormone Level	
	Suppression (glucose load)	Sharp drop in serum GH
Prolactin	Unstimulated	<20 ng/ml serum (>150 ng/ml - most likely tumor)
	Stimulation (thyroid-releasing hormone (TRH), chlorpromazine, dopamine)	Test not helpful
	Suppression	Test not helpful
Adreno-cortico-tropin (ACTH)	Unstimulated	2-15 ng/100 ml serum
	Stimulation (metyrapone, hypoglycemia)	Urine 17-hydroxycortico-steroids twice basal level; ACTH twice basal level
	Suppression (24-hr dexamethasone suppression)	Urine 17-hydroxy-corticosteroids <2.0 mg
	11 p.m.-1 mg dexamethasone	Plasma serum cortisol suppressed
Thyroid-stimulating hormone (TSH)	Unstimulated	0.5-10 microunits/ml serum
	Stimulated (TRH)	Twice unstimulated level
	Plasma-free T4	5-12 ng/ml
Follicular-stimulating hormone (FSH)	Unstimulated	Adult male 4-40 mIU/ml serum Adult female: Premeno-pausal: 5-30 mIU/ml serum Postmenopausal: 30-200 mIU/ml serum
	Stimulated (clomiphene)	1.2 x basal FSH
	Gonadotropic-releasing hormone	Not reliable

Table 6.1. (cont'd)

Hormone		Normal Hormone Level
Luteinizing Hormone (LH)	Unstimulated	Adult male 3-30 mIU/ml serum Adult female: Premenopausal: 5-100 mIU/ml serum Postmenopausal: 0-90 mIU/ml serum
	Stimulated (clomiphene)	1.3 x basal LH

REFERENCES

Black P: Brain metastasis: current status and recommended guidelines for management. Neurosurgery 5:617-631, 1979.

Burger PC, Vogel SF: Surgical Pathology of the Nervous System and Its Coverings, ed 2. New York, John Wiley & Sons, 1982.

Christy JH, Tindall GT: Endocrinologic diagnosis of pituitary tumor: indications for surgery and pre- and postoperative management. Clin Neurosurg 24:151-166, 1977.

Hart RG, and Davenport J: Diagnosis of acoustic neuroma. Neurosurgery 9:450-463, 1981.

Hildebrand J, Brihaye J: Chemotherapy of brain tumors. Adv Tech Stand Neurosurg 5:52-91, 1978.

Quest DO: Meningiomas: an update. Neurosurgery 3:219-225, 1978.

Sheline GE: Radiation therapy of brain tumors. Cancer 39:873-881, 1977.

Walker MD, Alexander Jr E, Hunt WE, et al: Evaluation of BCNU and/or radiotherapy in the treatment of anaplastic gliomas: a cooperative clinical trial. J Neurosurg 49:333-343, 1978.

Chapter 7

Stroke

The cerebral circulation, diagrammed in Figure 7.1, carries 800 ml of blood per minute, 80% of which flows through the carotid arteries. The circle of Willis, when fully developed, provides collateral blood flow to areas of the brain supplied by a compromised carotid or vertebral artery. Collateral flow can also be supplied through anastomoses with the external carotid artery.

Atherosclerosis, the primary cause of vascular occlusion, is most prevalent at the bifurcations of blood vessels. The origin of the internal carotid artery, just distal to the bifurcation of the common carotid artery, is the most common place for atherosclerosis to occur. The thrombosis of a badly stenosed lumen or hemorrhage into an atherosclerotic plaque may cause sudden vessel occlusion.

Subclavian steal results from an occlusion of the subclavian artery at its origin. Demand for blood in the distal subclavian artery is met by retrograde flow down the ipsilateral vertebral artery which steals blood from the circle of Willis. Most patients with this condition are asymptomatic, but a minority will manifest vertebrobasilar insufficiency (dizziness, syncope, visual disturbance) and arm ischemia (arm pain, fatigue, paresthesias) which are exacerbated by exercising the arm. The radial pulse of the affected arm is diminished.

Cerebrovascular disease is the third leading cause of death in the industrial world. Approximately 1.5 per 1,000 persons in the United States suffer from cerebral infarction each year. "Stroke" is a nonspecific term used for an acute neurological deficit resulting from vascular disease. Stroke is also used in a more specific sense to mean infarction of a portion of the brain. The differentiation of infarction from an intracranial mass lesion is not always simple and requires a firm knowledge of typical syndromes associated with infarction (Table 7.1).

A. Ischemic Disease

   1. Transient Ischemic Attacks (TIAs)

      Transient ischemic attacks (TIAs) are transient neurological deficits such as hemiparesis, monocular blindness, or sensory loss which last from minutes to no more than 24 hours. In between attacks, the patient has no residual deficit.

a. The neurological deficit reflects the distribution of the transient ischemia.

    i. TIAs in the carotid distribution: Amaurosis fugax (transient monocular blindness; the patient classically reports that the onset of his visual loss is like a shade coming down over his eye) or cortical deficits (e.g., hemiparesis, dysphasia, hemisensory deficit).

    ii. TIAs in the vertebrobasilar distribution: Homonymous field defect (e.g., graying of vision, scintillating scotomas), diplopia, dizziness, dysarthria, staggering of gait, vertigo, or brief loss of consciousness. Long-standing dizziness without other neurological problems is rarely a presentation of posterior circulation TIAs.

b. TIAs are thought to result from focal cerebral hypoperfusion or emboli originating in the carotid arteries, aorta, or heart.

c. Focal seizures, migraine attacks, or systemic diseases (e.g., hypoglycemia associated with diabetes mellitus, cardiac arrhythmias) may also be responsible for transient neurological deficits.

d. Anterior circulation TIAs resolve spontaneously in one-third of cases, persist in one-third of cases, and progress to stroke in one-third of cases. Posterior circulation TIAs are less prone to progress to stroke.

e. Cerebral artery occlusion is preceded by at least one TIA in 60% of cases.

2. Thrombotic Infarction

The neurological deficit associated with a thrombotic infarction usually evolves within a few hours. The deficit frequently occurs during sleep, but occasionally the neurological deficit may evolve over hours or days, mimicking an expanding mass lesion. Thrombosis most often involves the large extracranial vessels, such as the internal carotid artery.

a. Clinical picture:

    i. Approximately 60% of thrombotic infarctions are preceded by a TIA.

ii. The patient may have symptoms of generalized
     atherosclerosis, e.g., angina pectoris, intermit-
     tent claudication.

iii. The neurological deficit is confined to the distri-
     bution of the artery involved (see Table 7.1).

iv. The patient may have signs of atherosclerotic
     disease, e.g., diminished distal pulses, bruits
     over large blood vessels, and retinal changes.
     Special attention should be paid to bruits heard
     over the carotid arteries and to diminished super-
     ficial temporal pulses.

Table 7.1.
Cerebral Circulation

Anterior Cerebral Artery	All signs contralateral
Distal occlusion	Paralysis opposite leg Cortical sensory deficit most marked in the leg With bilateral lesions: Incontinence Abulia - slow mentation Grasp and suck reflexes
Proximal occlusion	All of the above plus: Facial and proximal arm weakness Frontal ataxia
Middle Cerebral Artery	All signs contralateral
General	Hemiplegia (face and arm greater than leg) Cortical sensory deficit Homonymous hemianopsia Transient paralysis of conjugate gaze
Dominant hemisphere	Broca's aphasia-paucity of speech Wernicke's aphasia-- difficulty understand- ing written or spoken language Acalculia--difficulty with calculations

Table 7.1. (cont'd)

	Agraphia--difficulty writing Right-left confusion Finger agnosia
Nondominant hemisphere	Dressing apraxia Constructional apraxia Ignoring contralateral space
Posterior Cerebral Artery	All signs contralateral
Distal	Homonymous hemianopsia Alexia--inability to read Memory deficit
Proximal	Infarction of thalamus or upper midbrain
Brain Stem Strokes	Complex, well defined syndromes based on anatomical considerations: Ipsilateral cranial nerve palsies Cerebellar signs and/or Horner's syndrome Contralateral body findings of weakness and sensory loss

    b. Diagnosis:

        i. Lumbar puncture, which is dangerous when there is
            swelling of the infarcted tissue, may demonstrate a
            slightly elevated protein value and an increased
            number of white blood cells in the CSF.

        ii. An EEG may demonstrate focal slowing.

        iii. A CT scan may begin to demonstrate low-density
            areas as early as 12 hours after a thrombotic
            stroke. The low density of infarction is maximal
            at 36 hours. Unlike cerebral edema, this low
            density does not stop at the border between the
            white matter and the cortex. Enhancement along the
            cortex and basal ganglia may be seen in the second

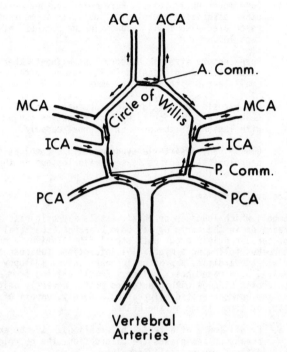

Figure 7.1. Anatomy of the cerebral circulation. ACA, anterior cerebral artery; MCA, middle cerebral artery; ICA, internal carotid artery; PCA, posterior cerebral artery; A. Comm., anterior communicating artery; P. Comm., posterior communicating artery.

                      week following infarction. Twenty percent of patients demonstrate significant cerebral swelling which can lead to uncal herniation.

        iv. Angiography may demonstrate an occluded vessel.

3. Lacunar Infarction

    Lacunes are small infarcts resulting from the thrombosis of small perforating blood vessels. These infarcts are associated with hypertensive vascular disease and may produce certain well defined neurological syndromes.

  a. Pure motor hemiparesis: Pure motor weakness without other associated neurological deficits is most often associated with small lacunes in the pons or internal capsule.

  b. Pure sensory stroke: Sensory loss without other associated neurological deficits is most often due to a small lesion within the thalamus.

  c. Leg paresis and ataxia: This unusual combination of weakness and difficulty with coordination can be seen with lesions in the pons or internal capsule.

  d. Clumsy hand dysarthria syndrome: This combination of neurological findings is seen with lesions in the upper third of the pons.

4. Cerebral Embolism

Emboli which lodge in cerebral vessels may originate in the heart or in the aorta or its main branches. Cerebral emboli of cardiac origin occur with atrial fibrillation, a mural thrombus following a myocardial infarction, subacute bacterial endocarditis, a prosthetic heart valve, a floppy mitral valve, or damaged heart valves. Emboli arising from atherosclerotic plaques within arteries most frequently originate at the common carotid bifurcation. Rarely, emboli of fat, air, or tumor lodge in the brain.

  a. Emboli lodge at arterial bifurcations. If the embolism breaks up and passes the bifurcation, the neurological deficit may partially resolve.

  b. The neurological deficit is abrupt in onset, non-progressive, and reflects the distribution of the artery occluded.

  c. The middle cerebral artery and its branches are the vessels most frequently affected.

  d. Hemorrhagic infarcts are pathognomonic for embolic events but are only seen in 30% of embolic infarctions.

  e. Seizures, which rarely occur in patients with thrombotic infarction, occur in 20% of patients with embolic strokes.

  f. Diagnosis:

    i. Although blood may be seen in the spinal fluid of patients who have suffered a hemorrhagic infarction, its absence does not rule out this condition.

ii. On the CT scan, the hemorrhagic infarct appears as a high-density central area surrounded by low density which fits the distribution of the involved artery.

iii. Angiography may demonstrate the abruptly occluded blood vessel which distally fills in a retrograde fashion.

5. Therapy of Ischemic Disease

a. Although attempts have been made to decrease the deficit associated with a stroke by increasing cerebral perfusion or altering cerebral metabolism, the efficacy of these methods remains to be proven. The best approach to stroke is prevention. A thorough investigation must be conducted to discover the source of a patient's TIAs, including investigation of the heart for arrhythmias, valvular vegetations, mural and valvular thrombi, or abnormal valvular motion and evaluation of the extra- and intracranial vessels for stenosis and sources of emboli. This entails an EKG (including a 24- or 48-hour monitor to evaluate rhythm), an echocardiogram, and an angiogram of the aortic arch and the carotid and vertebral arteries.

b. Although various authors have advocated the acute removal of an embolism or cerebral revascularization within the first 6 hours of stroke, the efficacy of this therapy remains to be proven.

c. Avoid postural changes which may precipitate hypotension. Do not use hypotensive agents in the acute poststroke period.

d. Drugs which decrease platelet adhesiveness such as aspirin or possibly dipyridamole (Persantine) appear to be of benefit in reducing the incidence of stroke in patients who have TIAs.

e. Anticoagulants are used to avoid the progression of TIAs to stroke, to arrest an evolving thrombotic infarction, or to prevent the thrombosis of a severely narrowed artery prior to surgical correction of the stenosis.

i. Heparin: Loading dose, 10,000 units over 15 minutes. Maintenance; 200-350 units per kg in 5% dextrose in water every 12 hours to run continuously. The rate of infusion should be adjusted to keep the partial thromboplastin time (PTT) 2-2.5 times normal (80-100 seconds).

      ii. Warfarin sodium: 2.5-10 mg, p.o., every day.
           Adjust dose so that prothrombin time is 1.5-2 times
           the control.

  f. Patients who have symptoms referable to the territory of
     the internal carotid artery concomitant with a high-
     grade stenosis or ulcerated plaque at the origin of that
     artery are best treated by carotid endarterectomy. This
     procedure entails opening the carotid artery at the site
     of the lesion and dissecting out its athromatous intima.
     Carotid TIAs most frequently are associated with disease
     at the level of the common carotid bifurcation. Endar-
     terectomy is only of benefit when the vessel lumen is at
     least partially patent and is almost never indicated
     after the internal carotid artery has become completely
     occluded. When the carotid is completely occluded, the
     thrombus extends up to the carotid siphon out of the
     reach of the surgeon.

  g. Cerebral blood flow can be enhanced by anastomosing a
     branch of the external carotid artery to a branch of the
     internal carotid artery distal to the occlusion. This
     is most often accomplished by anastomosing the super-
     ficial temporal artery or occipital artery to a branch
     of the middle cerebral artery. The efficacy of extra-
     cranial to intracranial bypass surgery is currently
     being evaluated.

  h. Physical therapy should be initiated to avoid contrac-
     tures in paralyzed limbs.

  i. Following the immediate poststroke period, attention
     should be turned to controlling hypertension, diabetes
     mellitus, hyperlipidemia, and other risk factors.

B. Hypertensive Intracranial Hemorrhage

Hypertensive hemorrhage within the parenchyma of the brain presents as a rapid loss of neurological function. General physical
examination reveals findings consistent with long-standing hypertension. Massive hypertensive hemorrhages may dissect into the
ventricles and subarachnoid spaces. The hemorrhage most frequently originates in the putamen or external capsule and dissects into
the ventricle or the frontal or temporal lobe.

  1. Types

     a. Putamental hemorrhage presents with a contralateral
        motor and sensory deficit because of involvement of the
        posterior internal capsule. The pupils are reactive to

light, but the eyes deviate toward the side of the
lesion. If the blood treks into the ventricles, the
patient may suffer sudden loss of consciousness. Brain
stem reflexes remain normal prior to uncal herniation.

b. Thalamic hemorrhage presents with a more profound
sensory loss than motor loss. Because of pressure on
the midbrain, the patient may manifest a Parinaud's
syndrome with eyes looking down, impairment of upward
gaze, small pupils, and poor pupillary reaction to
light.

c. Subcortical hemorrhages of hypertensive origin usually
occur in the posterior hemisphere at the gray-white
junction.

d. Pontine hemorrhage presents with headache associated
with nausea and vomiting. The patient loses
consciousness and on examination is found to have
quadriparesis, decerebrate posturing, loss of
extraocular movements, and pinpoint pupils.

e. Cerebellar hemorrhage most often presents with headache,
nausea, and vomiting. The cerebellar deficit is mild,
and gait ataxia predominates. As the brain stem is
compressed, the patient will develop difficulty with
lateral gaze or a sixth or seventh nerve palsy. Loss of
consciousness and Babinski signs occur late in the
evolution.

2. Treatment

The best treatment for a hypertensive hemorrhage is prevention with medical control of blood pressure. Supratentorial
hemorrhages are usually devastating. Surgical treatment is
reserved for the patient with an easily accessible hemorrhage, who manifests a deterioration in the level of consciousness. On the other hand, the evacuation of a cerebellar hemorrhage is lifesaving and is performed as a medical
emergency. If the hemorrhage is evacuated before the patient
loses consciousness, good results can be anticipated.
Cerebellar infarction can also present as a posterior fossa
mass necessitating emergency surgical decompression.

Table 7.2.
Evaluation of Stroke

---

1. History
    Previous TIAs, rate of progression, risk factors, possible
    contributing diseases.

2. Physical Examination
    Location of the lesion, associated mass effect, signs of
    hypertension, peripheral emboli, peripheral bruits.

3. Radiological Examination
    Location of the lesion, concomitant hemorrhage, intracranial
    mass effect, carotid atherosclerosis, valvular heart disease,
    other sources of emboli, vessel occlusion.

REFERENCES

Barnett HJM: Pathogenesis of transient ischemic attacks. In
Scheinberg P: Cerebrovascular Diseases: Tenth Princeton Conference.
New York, Raven Press, 1976, pp 1-21.

Ferguson GG: Extracranial carotid artery surgery. Clin
Neurosurg 29:543-574, 1982.

Fisher CM: Clinical syndromes in cerebral thrombosis,
hypertensive hemorrhage, and ruptured saccular aneurysm. Clin
Neurosurg 22:117-147, 1975.

Fisher CM: Lacunar strokes and infarcts: a review. Neurology
(NY) 32:871-876, 1982.

Peerless SJ: Techniques of cerebral revascularization. Clin
Neurosurg 23:258-269, 1976.

Peerless SJ, McCormick CW: Microsurgery for Cerebral
Ischemia. New York, Springer-Verlag, 1978.

Sundt TM Jr, Houser OW, Sharbrough FW, et al:
Carotid endarterectomy: results, complications, and monitoring
techniques. Adv Neurol 16:97-119, 1977.

Tew JM: Techniques of supratentorial cerebral revascularization.
Clin Neurosurg 26:330-345, 1979.

The Canadian Cooperative Study Group: A randomized trial of
aspirin and sulfinpyrazone in threatened stroke. N Engl J Med
299:53-59, 1978.

Toole JF, Yuson CP, Janeway R, et al: Transient ischemic
attacks: a prospective study of 225 patients. Neurology
(Minneap) 28:746-753, 1978.

Yatsu FM: Stroke: acute medical therapy of stroke. Stroke
13:524-526, 1982.

Chapter 8

Subarachnoid Hemorrhage

A. Spontaneous (Nontraumatic) Subarachnoid Hemorrhage

    1. Symptoms:

        a. The patient notes the sudden onset of a severe headache which persists for days and is refractory to common remedies.

        b. There may be concomitant nausea, vomiting, photophobia, seizure, or sudden loss of consciousness.

        c. The patient's level of consciousness may be depressed to varying degrees for varied periods of time.

        d. Rarely the patient may develop back and radicular leg pain as blood accumulates in the spinal canal.

    2. Signs:

        a. Physical examination reveals meningismus and a positive Kernig's sign.

        b. Globular subhyaloid hemorrhages, small scattered retinal hemorrhages, and papilledema may be seen on funduscopic examination.

        c. A focal neurological deficit indicates concomitant parenchymal damage.

    3. Laboratory investigations:

        a. Fever, leukocytosis, and an elevated blood pressure are not unusual.

        b. CT scan may reveal blood in one or more cisterns or focal areas of hemorrhage.

        c. Lumbar puncture, which should not be performed when a large intraparenchymal hemorrhage is suspected, reveals red blood cells in the spinal fluid; the same degree of coloration of the CSF by blood persists through

several successively collected tubes. Most patients
with subarachnoid hemorrhage will initially have an
elevated CSF pressure. More than 6 hours after the
hemorrhage, the supernatant of the centrifuged spinal
fluid is xanthochromic. Iron can be detected in CSF
macrophages for the ensuing 4 months.

   d. Two-thirds of the patients with subarachnoid hemorrhage
       will have abnormalities demonstrated by angiography.

B. Aneurysms

   1. <u>Intracranial berry aneurysms</u> are thin-walled arterial
       outpouchings which usually occur at the branching points of
       major arteries at the base of the brain: 85% involve the
       anterior circle of Willis and its branches, and 15% involve
       the vertebral-basilar circulation. There is an increased
       incidence of berry aneurysms with Type III polycystic renal
       disease, coarctation of the aorta, and the Ehler-Danlos
       syndrome. Although aneurysms usually come to clinical
       attention because of subarachnoid hemorrhage, some do so by
       pressing on adjacent structures (Table 8.1). Prior to the
       devastating rupture of an aneurysm, there is often a "warning
       leak" with concomitant headache. Occasionally aneurysmal
       rupture may produce a subdural hematoma. The patient's
       clinical condition is graded as per Table 8.2.

Table 8.1.
Aneurysm Presenting as an Intracranial Mass

Location	Symptom
Internal carotid-posterior communicating artery junction	Third nerve palsy
Posterior cerebral-posterior communicating artery junction	Third nerve palsy
Internal carotid-ophthalmic artery junction	Monocular visual field deficit
Anterior communicating artery	Chiasmal syndrome
Giant aneurysm (>2.5 cm in diameter) in any location	Tumor mass

Table 8.2.
Hunt's Classification of Aneurysms*

---

0   Unruptured aneurysm

I   Asymptomatic, or minimal headache and slight nuchal rigidity

Ia   No acute meningeal or brain reaction but fixed neurological
      deficit

II   Moderate to severe headache, nuchal rigidity, no neurological
      deficit other than cranial nerve palsy

III   Drowsiness, confusion, or mild focal deficit

IV   Stupor, moderate to severe hemiparesis, possibly early
      decerebrate rigidity and vegetative disturbances

V   Deep coma, decerebrate rigidity, moribund appearance

---

*Place in next worse category if a serious systemic disease
(e.g., hypertensive cardiovascular disease, diabetes mellitus,
chronic obstructive pulmonary disease) or severe intracranial
arterial spasm is present.

   a. Common aneurysms:

       i.   Internal carotid-ophthalmic artery junction
            aneurysms are most common in females and are
            occasionally bilateral. They may come to clinical
            attention because of visual field deficits.

       ii. Internal carotid-posterior communicating artery
            junction aneurysms may present with a third nerve
            palsy. The third nerve palsy associated with an
            intracranial aneurysm may often be distinguished
            from that associated with diabetes mellitus because
            in the latter condition the pupil may be spared
            (i.e., not dilated).

       iii. Anterior communicating artery aneurysms may present
            as a loss of vision from compression of the optic
            chiasm. Rupture of this type of aneurysm may
            damage the hypothalamus.

       iv. Middle cerebral artery aneurysms may rupture into
            the brain parenchyma, producing hemiplegia,
            dysphasia, or hemianopsia.

  v. Basilar bifurcation aneurysms are the most common
      aneurysms found in the posterior circulation.

b. Diagnosis:

  i. A lumbar puncture performed after a "warning leak"
      will reward the physician with the presumptive
      diagnosis of an aneurysm prior to a devastating
      hemorrhage.

  ii. The definitive diagnosis is then made by
      angiography. Since 20% of patients harbor multiple
      aneurysms, the entire intracranial circulation must
      be studied.

  iii. A CT scan will frequently demonstrate subarachnoid
      hemorrhage and may even demonstrate the aneurysm.
      The CT scan is essential in revealing an associated
      intracerebral blood clot.

  iv. EKG abnormalities occur commonly in patients with
      subarachnoid hemorrhage; they include arrhythmias
      and changes indicative of myocardial ischemia or
      infarction. Pulmonary edema is sometimes
      encountered.

c. Prognosis:

  i. Previously unruptured aneurysms bleed at a rate of
      1-2.5% per year.

  ii. There appears to be a correlation of aneurysm size
      and propensity to rupture.

  iii. Each significant hemorrhage is accompanied by about
      a 45% mortality. Rebleeding poses the greatest
      danger to survivors, as 50% of ruptured aneurysms
      will bleed again within the next 6 months. The
      chances for a second hemorrhage are greatest during
      the 4 weeks after the initial rupture.

  iv. Patients with a higher clinical grade (Table 8.2)
      have a worse prognosis.

d. Delayed complications of subarachnoid hemorrhage

  i. Hydrocephalus. Communicating hydrocephalus occurs
      as a result of interference with CSF circulation
      and absorption by the subarachnoid blood. Although
      the hydrocephalus often resolves spontaneously, it
      may require shunting.

      ii. Inappropriate secretion of antidiuretic hormone: fluid retention with a decreased serum sodium concentration.

     iii. Cerebral vasospasm, the narrowing of intracranial arteries, is encountered in at least 35% of patients with subarachnoid hemorrhage from a ruptured aneurysm. It occurs most frequently 4-14 days after the aneurysm ruptures. Cerebral vasospasm is often associated with a decline in neurological function, usually on the basis of cerebral ischemia. The cause of symptomatic cerebral vasospasm remains obscure, but if it is untreated, it can lead to a stroke. Patients with large amounts of subarachnoid blood, as seen on the initial CT scan, are most likely to develop this complication. The only proven treatment is the elevation of intravascular volume and elevation of systemic blood pressure, which increase the risk of aneurysm rupture unless the aneurysm has already been isolated from the intracranial circulation surgically.

  e. Treatment

The definitive treatment of intracranial aneurysms is surgical. Most frequently the base of the aneurysm is ligated with a metal clip or a silk suture. Aneurysms which are not amenable to this treatment may be wrapped with muslin or coated with plastic. Aneurysms of the internal carotid artery are occasionally treated by the gradual occlusion of the cervical portion of the carotid artery in order to lower the pressure within the aneurysm. Because of the possibility of aggravating the ischemic effects of cerebral vasospasm, many surgeons delay surgery for 2 weeks. During this time, precautions are taken to avoid a sudden elevation in blood pressure which may rupture the aneurysm. However, restrictions should not be so strict that the patient becomes anxious.

      i. Bed rest, quiet room, dimmed lights to avoid photophobia.

      ii. Limited visitation.

     iii. Stool softeners.

     iv. Nothing per rectum.

      v. Avoid urinary retention.

vi. Mild sedative to suppress anxiety but not to change mental status.

vii. Precautions to keep a confused patient from falling out of bed.

viii. Diet - avoid very hot or very cold fluids.

ix. Vital signs - frequent neurological assessments are especially important during the period when vasospasm is most likely to occur.

x. Medications.

1) Antifibrinolytic agents such as ε-aminocaproic acid (Amicar, 3 g i.v. q 2 h given by continuous infusion for 2 weeks), have been demonstrated to diminish the likelihood of a second hemorrhage during the first 2 weeks following aneurysm rupture.

2) Antihypertensive medications must be used with caution. Acute arterial hypertension frequently accompanies a subarachnoid hemorrhage. Lowering the blood pressure may precipitate or worsen neurological deficits that are due to ischemia.

xi. Vasospasm is treated by increasing the patient's blood volume with colloid solutions or blood (the patient's hematocrit should be approximately 35%). This is best monitored with a Swan-Ganz catheter. Hypertensive agents such as dopamine are sometimes used.

xii. Hydrocephalus may be treated temporarily by draining CSF (slowly). Because lowering the intracranial pressure may precipitate hemorrhage from the aneurysm, this procedure is only done on patients who are severely compromised by their hydrocephalus.

2. Atherosclerotic aneurysms are ectatic dilatations of atherosclerotic intracranial vessels. These aneurysms, which most frequently involve the vertebral-basilar system, seldom bleed but come to attention by pressing adjacent structures such as cranial nerves. These aneurysms may thrombose, causing infarction.

3. Mycotic aneurysms arise from inflamed blood vessels. They can arise in the face of bacterial endocarditis, sepsis, or meningitis. These aneurysms may be multiple and most often

appear on the distal branches of intracranial arteries (especially the middle cerebral artery). They are probably best treated by surgical obliteration.

C. Vascular Malformations

1. Vascular malformations usually come to medical attention because of parenchymal and perhaps subarachnoid or intraventricular hemorrhage. They can also present with a seizure disorder, headaches, or cerebral ischemia. Pathological examination differentiates vascular malformations into four categories.

    a. Telangiectasias are capillary tufts which are separated by normal brain. They occur most frequently in the pons and seldom bleed.

    b. Cavernous angiomas are composed of closely packed small sinusoidal vessels without intervening parenchyma.

    c. Arteriovenous malformations (AVMs) are composed of varying sized arteries and veins which are separated by gliotic hemosiderin-laden parenchyma.

    d. Venous angiomas are characterized by an extensive venous network separated by normal parenchyma.

2. Prognosis

    Vascular malformations are more benign than aneurysms. The mortality from the rupture of an arteriovenous malformation increases from about 10% with the first bleeding episode to about 20% with the third.

Table 8.3.
Prognosis for AVM

Presentation	Rebleed Rate
Seizures, headache, etc. (but no bleeding)	1%/yr (25% in 15 yr)
Single hemorrhage	3-4%/yr (25% in 4 yr)
Two hemorrhages	25% in 1 yr

3. Definitive visualization of the lesion is made by angiography, but the CT scan will demonstrate many of these lesions and will also reveal any associated hemorrhage.

4. Therapy

    a. Primary surgical excision.

    b. Embolization with an agent such as Gelfoam, beads, or cyanoacrylate.

    c. Focused radiotherapy may sclerose some lesions.

    d. Ligation of feeding vessels only is of limited value.

D. Subarachnoid Hemorrhage of Other Causes

    1. Spontaneous subarachnoid hemorrhage not associated with vascular anomalies may in some cases be due to hypertensive vascular disease, a brain tumor, cerebral vasculitis, a blood dyscrasia, anticoagulation therapy, meningitis, syphilis, encephalitis, systemic lupus erythematosis, polyarteritis nodosa, etc. In general, however, patients with subarachnoid hemorrhage who do not have an aneurysm or AVM on angiography have a good prognosis.

    2. Sturge-Weber disease is characterized by a port wine nevus of the face and a meningeal angioma involving the pia and the arachnoid (usually in the occipital region). Clinical manifestations include mental retardation, epilepsy, glaucoma, homonymous hemianopsia, and sometimes hemiplegia. Subarachnoid hemorrhage almost never occurs. X-ray films of the skull usually demonstrate the characteristic intracranial calcifications.

REFERENCES

Drake CG: Management of cerebral aneurysms. Stroke 12:273-283, 1981.

Peerless SJ: Pre- and postoperative management of cerebral aneurysms. Clin Neurosurg 26:209-231, 1979.

Rhoton AL Jr, Saeki N, Perlmutter D, et al: Microscopic anatomy of common aneurysm sites. Clin Neurosurg 26:248-306, 1979.

Sundt TM Jr and Whisnant JP: Subarachnoid hemorrhage from intracranial aneurysms: surgical management and natural history of disease. N Engl J Med 299:116-122, 1978.

Chapter 9

Pediatric Neurosurgery

A. Head Enlargement

The head reaches 80% of its adult circumference by the time that the child is 1 year of age. The normal increase in the size of the skull reflects the enlargement of the brain, which reaches 50% of its adult weight by 1 year of age. An abnormally rapid increase in the growth of the head, as seen when the head circumference is mapped on standard growth charts, reflects an abnormal increase in intracranial contents.

In infants with increased intracranial pressure, the anterior fontanelle becomes enlarged and tense, losing its normal pulsations. X-ray films may demonstrate an abnormally large separation of the sutures or prominent convolutional markings ("beaten silver" pattern). With increased intracranial pressure, the child may become irritable or feed poorly. Developmental milestones may be reached more slowly or those previously obtained may be lost. The infant may have noticeable paralysis of upward gaze and appear to be looking down chronically, the "setting sun" sign. Percussion of the skull with split sutures reveals the "cracked pot" sign.

Head enlargement may result from various conditions, including hydrocephalus, subdural fluid collections, intracranial tumors and cysts, achondroplasia, and neuronal storage disease.

1. Constitutional macrocrania is a familial head enlargement with a normal rate of head growth. Neurological examination does not reveal signs of increased intracranial pressure.

2. Hydrocephalus is defined as a disproportionate enlargement of part or all of the cerebral ventricular system, concomitant with an increase in the amount of CSF within the head.

    a. Hydrocephalus usually results from obstruction of the normal flow of CSF and only rarely from CSF overproduction as occurs with a choroid plexus papilloma. Obstruction to CSF flow may be due to a congenital malformation (e.g., stenosis of the aqueduct), an intracranial neoplasm, or subarachnoid inflammation from meningitis or subarachnoid hemorrhage.

b. Periodic elevations in CSF pressure (i.e., pressure
    waves) may be superimposed on a baseline normal
    pressure, leading to ventricular enlargement. For this
    reason, a single spinal tap may not reveal the increased
    pressure which is responsible for the hydrocephalus.

c. Infants with hydrocephalus may demonstrate signs of
    increased intracranial pressure and bilateral frontal
    prominence of the head. Older patients may present with
    symptoms of increased intracranial pressure or with
    gait disturbance, urinary incontinence, and progressive
    dementia.

d. The diagnosis of hydrocephalus:

    i.   CT scan or ultrasound sonogram demonstrates ven-
         tricular enlargement.

    ii. Cerebrospinal fluid pressure may be increased.

    iii. Diffuse transillumination of the head is seen with
         severe hydrocephalus.

e. Classification of hydrocephalus

    i.   Communicating hydrocephalus indicates obstruction
         of CSF flow in the subarachnoid cisterns or poor
         CSF absorption at the Pacchionian granulations.
         The ventricles all communicate and are all
         enlarged.

    ii. Noncommunicating hydrocephalus implies that the
         obstruction of CSF flow is within the ventricular
         system.

    iii. Normal pressure hydrocephalus is communicating
         hydrocephalus which occurs (typically in an adult)
         in the face of obstensibly normal CSF pressure.
         This type of hydrocephalus most likely results from
         periodic waves of increased pressure.

    iv. Hydrocephalus ex vacuo refers to the ventricular
         enlargement which results from the loss of brain
         parenchyma rather than from the overproduction or
         underabsorption of CSF or an obstruction to CSF
         flow.

f. Causes of hydrocephalus

    i.   Aqueductal stenosis may result from gliosis around
         the aqueduct of Sylvius in response to an inflamma-
         tory process or may be the result of a congenital

malformation of the aqueduct. Diagnostic studies demonstrate enlargement of the lateral and third ventricles but not of the fourth ventricle.

ii. The Dandy-Walker syndrome consists of a small malformed cerebellum, a large posterior fossa cyst in communication with the fourth ventricle, and obstruction to the flow of CSF from the fourth ventricle to the subarachnoid cisterns. Enlargement of the posterior fossa results in a prominent occiput.

iii. Intracranial tumors or cysts may deform the normal CSF pathways, obstructing the flow of spinal fluid. This is especially common with a medulloblastoma or ependymoma of the fourth ventricle.

iv. Vein of Galen aneurysms are vascular malformations which may deform the aqueduct and cause hydrocephalus. These lesions also may present with congestive heart failure or subarachnoid hemorrhage.

v.   Leptomeningeal inflammation resulting from infection or subarachnoid hemorrhage may cause adhesions and obstruction of the subarachnoid cisterns and damage to the Pacchionian granulations.

vi. Periventricular hemorrhage extending into the ventricles is most likely to occur in premature infants subjected to a hypoxic-ischemic insult (e.g., the respiratory distress syndrome). These children must be monitored for the development of hydrocephalus.

g. Treatment of hydrocephalus consists of shunting the CSF to a cavity from which it can be absorbed. Prophylactic antibiotics (e.g., 40 mg per kg of cephalothin i.v. during the induction of anesthesia and 40 mg per kg i.v., q 6 h x 3 days postoperatively, as well as direct shunt injections) have been shown to be of benefit in reducing the postoperative infection rate.

Types of shunts:

i.   A ventriculoatrial shunt diverts the CSF from the lateral ventricle to the right atrium of the heart. Complications include mechanical obstruction of the shunt (which may present as obtundation, nausea, and vomiting), infection, subdural hematomas, thromboembolism, shunt nephritis, cardiac

arrhythmias, bacterial endocarditis, pulmonary
emboli, vena cava thrombosis, and (rarely) cardiac
perforation.

ii. A ventriculoperitoneal shunt diverts the fluid to
the peritoneal cavity. Complications include shunt
obstruction, infection, subdural hematomas,
abdominal CSF pseudocysts, intestinal volvulus, and
perforation of the viscera.

iii. Third ventriculostomy is the surgical perforation
of the anterior wall of the third ventricle to
establish a communication between the ventricular
system and the subarachnoid cisterns. To be
effective, it requires that the patient be able to
absorb CSF from the subarachnoid spaces.

iv. Ventriculocisternostomy (Torkildsen shunt) entails
passing a shunt tube(s) from one or both of the
lateral ventricles to the upper cervical
subarachnoid space. This bypasses an occluded
aqueduct of Sylvius.

v. Lumbar-peritoneal shunting is the procedure of
choice for refractory pseudotumor cerebri. Scoliosis may be a late complication.

3. Arachnoid cysts occur most frequently in the middle fossa,
over the cerebral convexity, in the suprasellar area, or over
the surface of the cerebellum. They present in infancy as
head enlargement or later in life as an intracranial mass.
The cyst is composed of arachnoid and filled with CSF.
Treatment consists of excising the cyst, fenestrating its
wall so that it communicates with a subarachnoid cistern or
ventricle, or shunting it as one would shunt a hydrocephalic
ventricle.

4. Subdural fluid collections resulting from hematoma or
effusion are another cause of macrocephaly.

a. Subdural hematomas are most frequently the consequence
of head trauma. In the newborn, subdural hematomas
result from trauma at the time of delivery, perhaps
complicated by vitamin K deficiency, coagulopathy, and
perinatal asphyxia.

i. Subdural hematomas in infants tend to be bilateral
and present with seizures, lethargy, irritability,
retarded development, low-grade fever, anemia,
subhyaloid hemorrhages, and symptoms and signs of
increased intracranial pressure.

      ii. The head demonstrates biparietal enlargement.

     iii. Child abuse should be considered.

     iv. In children over 2 years of age, subdural hematomas tend to be unilateral and behave like their adult counterparts. As in adults, these blood collections may become encapsulated and enlarge if left untreated.

     v. The diagnosis is best established by CT scan. A long-standing subdural hematoma will cause an enlargement of the middle fossa detectable on plain roentgenograms.

     vi. Chronic subdural hematomas may be diagnosed in infants by subdural taps done through the lateral margins of the open anterior fontanelle or through the coronal sutures.

  b. Subdural effusions occur as a complication of bacterial meningitis, most often due to Haemophilus influenzae. They occur during the first 2 years of life and usually are sterile. The diagnosis is made by CT scan or supratentorial transillumination. Enlarging or persistent collections are drained by subdural taps in order to avoid the formation of encapsulated fluid collections.

    Treatment of subdural collections in infants consists of daily subdural taps. If the fluid fails to resolve after 2 weeks, it may be drained externally for 2 days or shunted from the subdural cavity to the peritoneal or pleural space. Rarely, craniotomy with removal of membranes will be necessary.

B. Malformations at the Craniovertebral Junction

  1. The Chiari Type I malformation is the chronic displacement of the cerebellar tonsils into the upper cervical spinal canal. This malformation may be associated with syringomyelia. Adults most commonly present with occipital or cervical pain but may present with visual dysfunction (e.g., downbeating nystagmus), exertional headaches, lower cranial nerve palsies, ataxia, signs of spinal cord compression (e.g., corticospinal and sensory deficits), or symptoms of a central cord syndrome.

  2. The Chiari Type II malformation (Arnold-Chiari malformation) is the displacement of the cerebellar vermis into the cervical canal, caudal displacement of the pons and medulla, and elongation of the fourth ventricle. Concomitant with

this caudal displacement of the hindbrain, there may be
"beaking" of the quadrigeminal plate, aqueductal stenosis,
polymicrogyria, enlargement of the massa intermedia, syringomyelia, and cortical heterotopias. This often presents as
hydrocephalus. Plain skull films demonstrate a small
posterior fossa and an enlarged foramen magnum. The CT scan
may demonstrate craniolacunia (which disappears by 6 months
of age), petrous scalloping, foramen magnum enlargement,
hypoplasia of the falx cerebri and tentorium, beaking of the
quadrigeminal plate, hydrocephalus, malformation of the
frontal horns as well as caudal displacement of the fourth
ventricle, inferior vermis, and medulla.

3. Bony malformations

    a. Platybasia is flattening of the base of the skull.

    b. Basilar impression, the upward migration of the
       cervical spine into the base of the skull, may be
       developmental in origin or the result of Paget's
       disease, rickets, osteomalacia, or hyperparathyroidism.

    c. Assimilation of the atlas is the fusion of the atlas to
       the occiput.

4. Neurological examination may reveal signs of a foramen magnum
syndrome, downgaze nystagmus, cerebellar dysfunction,
spasticity, central cord syndrome, or bulbar palsy.

C. Spinal Dysraphism

1. Vertebral anomalies

Vertebral bodies may be split in the sagittal or coronal
direction. A sagittally cleft vertebra may be associated
with a meningocele, a myelomeningocele, diastematomyelia, or
visceral anomalies. Hemivertebrae result from failure of
one-half of the vertebral body to form. Spine films
demonstrate a laterally displaced triangular wedge of bone
between two normal vertebral bodies.

Spina bifida occulta refers to a lack of fusion of a neural
arch in a patient in whom this defect is not suspected from
physical examination alone. When it is present, this abnormality commonly involves the L5 or S1 vertebra, and it is
usually asymptomatic.

2. Lipomyelomeningocele usually presents as a subcutaneous mass
of fatty tissue which passes intradurally and is continuous
with the conus medullaris. The conus is usually tethered
down in the lower lumbar area. Surgical repair must include

untethering the cord, debulking the fat, and closing the dura.

3. A myelomeningocele is the protrusion of neural elements through a vertebral defect (usually posteriorly) into a sac where they are covered to a variable degree by meninges and skin. The neural elements are adherent to this covering. The disorder most frequently involves the lumbar spine. In families where one child is affected, there is an increased risk of the disorder occurring in siblings. Myelomeningoceles are almost always associated with an Arnold-Chiari defect and are frequently associated with hydrocephalus and other congenital anomalies. Because of the devastating effects of meningitis, the defect should be closed within 24 hours after birth if possible.

4. A _meningocele_ is a protrusion of meninges (devoid of accompanying nervous elements) through a defect in the spine. Such protrusions most frequently occur posteriorly in the lumbosacral region but can protrude anteriorly or laterally, especially in the thoracic region. Unlike myelomeningoceles, they are not associated with the Arnold-Chiari malformation or hydrocephalus. Myelography and/or spinal CT scanning is necessary to determine the position of the normal neural elements. Plain x-ray films of the spine demonstrate only the bony defects.

5. Occult Dysraphic States

    Occult dysraphic states are a series of spinal and intraspinal abnormalities that are not directly apparent to inspection of the external surface of the body. Its most benign form is spina bifida occulta, a failure of the posterior bony elements of the spine to fuse. More sinister forms may come to attention because of a cutaneous abnormality overlying the spine such as a port wine stain, dimple, sinus tract, hairy patch, or subcutaneous lipoma. Although the intraspinal abnormality may be silent at birth, the child may develop a gait abnormality, back pain, scoliosis, a foot deformity, incontinence, sensory loss in the saddle area, or leg weakness as he matures. Roentgenograms of the spine may reveal a hemivertebra or incomplete fusion of the neural arch. Myelography is necessary to diagnose most of the abnormalities definitively; spinal CT scanning is also of value.

    Hypertrophy of the filum terminale is associated with tethering of the conus of the spinal cord below its normal position. The child usually comes to attention between the ages of 5 and 10 years. Treatment consists of dividing the hypertrophied filum terminale.

Diastematomyelia is the division of the spinal cord into two
parallel portions over one or more spinal segments. Often
the two portions are separated by an osseous or fibrous
septum which lies in the sagittal plane. Although this
disorder is occasionally associated with a myelomeningocele,
it is rarely associated with hydrocephalus. Plain x-ray
films may demonstrate widening of the neural canal,
associated vertebral anomalies, and at times the bony spur
itself. Myelography, with or without spinal CT scanning, is
usually the definitive test. Unless found as an asymptomatic
lesion in an adult, this lesion should be removed
surgically to prevent the subsequent development or
progression of neurological or skeletal abnormalities.

A dermal sinus tract is an elongated epithelial-lined pouch
which empties through a small hole in the skin, usually in
the midline in the sacral or lower lumbar region. The
cul-de-sac may extend anywhere from the subcutaneous tissue
to the conus of the spinal cord. Symptoms are caused by an
associated dermoid or epidermoid tumor within the conus or
spinal canal, or by infection which enters through this
epithelial lined passageway. A similar dermal sinus may trek
from the suboccipital area into the fourth ventricle.

Neurenteric cysts result from errors in the normal
embryological interrelationships of the endoderm, notochord,
and neural ectoderm. Such a cyst may occur within the spinal
canal, usually in the low cervical or thoracic area. It acts
as a compressive mass, impinging on the spinal cord or
enlarging within the cord.

D. Craniosynostosis

Craniosynostosis, the premature closure of one or more cranial
sutures, produces a deformity of the infant's skull which becomes
more prominent as the skull enlarges. This differs from microcephaly where the small brain provides no impetus for the skull to
grow. Although occasionally familial and rarely secondary to
trauma or a metabolic abnormality, this condition is usually
idiopathic. Unless more than one suture is involved, craniosynostosis presents primarily a cosmetic problem.

Because the infant's skull reaches 80% of its adult size by the
end of the first year, surgical release of the fused suture(s)
must be done early to change the shape of the head effectively.
The ideal time for repair is at 4-6 weeks of life. In older
children, more extensive plastic surgery is necessary.

1. <u>Sagittal synostosis</u> (scaphocephaly) causes the child's head to be elongated in its fronto-occipital dimensions. This is the most common form of craniosynostosis; 80% of the patients with this condition are male.

2. <u>Coronal synostosis</u> (brachycephaly) is occasionally familial and is sometimes associated with Crouzon's or Apert's syndrome. It causes the anterior part of the calvarium to be short and wide, with a high flat forehead and shallow orbits. Coronal synostosis may be unilateral, causing an asymmetry of the forehead and orbit.

3. <u>Lambdoidal synostosis</u> is rare and causes flattening of the occiput on one or both sides.

4. <u>Metopic synostosis</u> (trigonocephaly) produces narrowing of the forehead with a prominent sagittal ridge.

5. <u>Oxycephaphy</u> (tower skull) results from the premature closure of all sutures. If not corrected, increased intracranial pressure, visual loss (from optic atrophy), mental retardation, and other serious sequelae occur.

REFERENCES

Anderson FM: Occult spinal dysraphism: a series of 73 cases. <u>Pediatrics</u> 55:826-835, 1975.

Black PM: Idiopathic normal-pressure hydrocephalus: results of shunting in 62 patients. <u>J Neurosurg</u> 52:371-377, 1980.

Golbus MS, Loughman WD, Epstein CJ, et al: Prenatal genetic diagnosis in 3000 amniocenteses. <u>N Engl J Med</u> 300:157-163, 1979.

Hahn JF, Jane JA: Craniosynostosis and related syndrome: pathogenesis and treatment. <u>Cleve Clin</u> 45:213-217, 1978.

Keucher TR, Mealey J: Long-term results after ventriculo-atrial and ventriculoperitoneal shunting for infantile hydro-cephalus. <u>J Neurosurg</u> 50:179-186, 1979.

McRae DL: Bony abnormalities at the cranio-spinal junction. <u>Clin Neurosurg</u> 16:356-375, 1969.

Milhorat TH: <u>Pediatric Neurosurgery</u>. Philadelphia, F A Davis, 1978.

Peach B: Arnold Chiari malformation: anatomic features of 20 cases. <u>Arch Neurol</u> 12:613-621, 1965.

Section of Pediatric Neurosurgery of the American Association of Neurological Surgeons: Pediatric Neurosurgery: Surgery of the Developing Nervous System. New York, Grune & Stratton, 1982.

Shillito J: Surgical approaches to spina bifida and myelomeningocele. Clin Neurosurg 20:114-133, 1973.

Spillane JD, Pallis C, Jones AM: Developmental abnormalities in the region of the foramen magnum. Brain 80:11-48, 1957.

Udvarhelyi GB, Epstein MH: The so called Dandy Walker syndrome: analysis of 12 operated cases. Childs Brain 1:158-182, 1975.

Chapter 10

The Spine

A. The Cervical Spine

   A systematic approach should be used when examining x-ray films of the cervical spine. If the patient is suspected of having sustained cervical trauma, the films should be taken before the patient is moved off of the ambulance stretcher or spine board (Fig. 10.1).

   1. Lateral Cervical Spine Films

      a. All seven vertebral bodies must be visualized for the study to be complete.

      b. Examination begins with an evaluation of the soft tissue. Edema, hematoma, tumor infiltration, or infection can cause widening of the soft tissue shadow in front of the vertebral column (see Table 10.1).

      c. The posterior borders of the vertebral bodies are aligned to form a smooth concave curve. This curve can be disrupted by traumatic lesions, degenerative arthritis, or rheumatoid arthritis.

      d. Adult vertebral bodies are rectangular, sharply outlined by cortical bone, and separated by radiolucent intervertebral discs. (The vertebral bodies of infants are oval.) Note any loss of vertebral body height, obscuration of cortical bone, or narrowing of the intervertebral disc.

      e. The right and left articular pillars are superimposed and have a trapezoid shape. A wedging of one articular pillar implies a compressive fracture, and lack of superimposition implies rotation of the spine.

      f. The spinous processes should be equally spaced and should fan out evenly on flexion of the spine.

CERVICAL SPINE

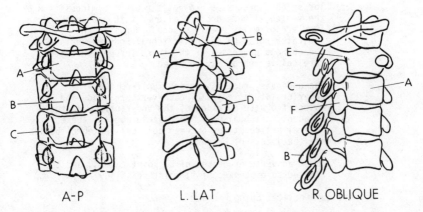

A-P   L. LAT   R. OBLIQUE

Figure 10.1 Cervical spine. A, vertebral body. B, posterior spinous process. C, articular pillar. D, lamina. E, pedicle. F, neural foramen.

Table 10.1.
Maximum Normal Cervical Soft Tissue Measurements

	Adults	Children
Posterior pharynx to anterior-inferior edge of C_2	7 mm	7 mm
Posterior trachea to anterior-inferior edge of C_6	22 mm	14 mm
Atlas to anterior dens	3 mm	5 mm

2. Anterior-Posterior Cervical Spine Films

    a. The lateral masses of the atlas should be equidistant from the odontoid process and directly above the superior articular facets of the axis.

    b. The odontoid process is centered over the body of the axis. A cartilaginous synchondrosis is present between the odontoid process and the body of the atlas until the age of 10 and should not be mistaken for a fracture.

    c. The spinous processes project through the midposition of the vertebral body and are aligned with one another. They are normally evenly spaced. Nonalignment indicates rotation of one vertebral body on another. The spinous processes of the third through the fifth cervical vertebrae may be bifed.

    d. The uncinate processes project up from the superior-lateral edges of each vertebral body and are associated with beveling of the undersurface of the adjacent vertebral body immediately above. These lateral articulations between cervical vertebral bodies are the joints of Luschka.

    e. The transverse processes of C7 point caudad, and the transverse processes of T1 point cephalad.

3. Oblique Cervical Spine Films

    a. The neural foramina are seen as ovals framed superiorly and inferiorly by the pedicles. Encroachment into a neural foramen by spondylotic ridges or fractured bony spicules is seen on this projection.

    b. The articular pillars appear as parallelograms. Their shape and alignment should be inspected.

    c. The ipsilateral laminae are seen on end and overlap as do the shingles on a roof. Loss of this shingling indicates disruption of the posterior articulation.

B. The Lumbar Spine (Fig. 10.2)

1. Lateral Lumbar Spine Films

    a. The vertebral body appears as a dense rectangle of cortical bone filled with coarse trabeculated bone.

    b. The neural foramina are seen between the pedicles.

LUMBAR SPINE

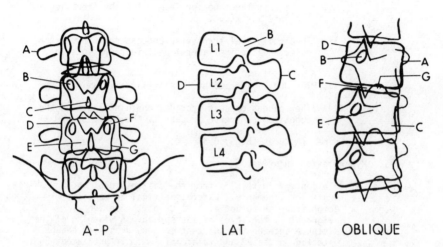

Figure 10.2. Lumbar spine. A, transverse process. B, pedicle.
C, posterior spinous process. D, vertebral body. E, lamina.
F, superior articular facet. G, inferior articular facet.

2. Anterior-Posterior (AP) Lumbar Spine Films

   a. The vertebral bodies are rectangular with sharply
       defined margins.

   b. The pedicles project as an oval over the lateral aspect
       of the vertebral body on each side. The pedicles may be
       obliterated by metastatic tumor or may be spread apart
       by a fracture.

   c. The superior and inferior facets are attached medially
       to the broad laminae to produce a pattern similar to the
       wings of a butterfly. The disruption of the articula-
       tion of adjacent facets may be the only sign of a
       dislocation.

       d. The spinous processes are centered in the midline and are evenly spaced. They form the body of the butterfly.

   3. Oblique Lumbar Spine Films

       a. The superimposed posterior elements form the "Scottie" dog. The components of the "Scottie" dog represent the following:

           i. The ear is the superior facet, and the front leg is the inferior facet.

          ii. The ipsilateral transverse process contributes the nose, and the ipsilateral pedicle represents the eye.

        iii. The body is formed by the ipsilateral lamina.

        iv. The spinous process provides the hind leg, and the opposite transverse process is the tail.

C. Cervical Spine Fractures (Fig. 10.3)

   1. Hyperflexion Injuries

       a. Flexion sprain results from the disruption of the posterior ligaments. Lateral cervical spine films demonstrate an abrupt alteration of the vertebral alignment at the level of the sprain. A widening of the distance between the adjacent spinous processes can be detected on the AP and lateral films. If untreated, 20% remain unstable.

       b. Bilateral locked facets are caused by disruption of ligamentous support and the anterior rotation of the inferior facet of the apophyseal joint up and over the superior facet. The lateral film demonstrates an anterior displacement of the vertebral body, and oblique films demonstrate the abnormal position of the facets. Unless there is a fracture of the vertebral ring, this injury is almost always associated with spinal cord damage.

       c. Unilateral locked facets occur when a single inferior facet rotates forward and over the tip of the superior facet. The oblique x-ray film demonstrates the disrupted posterior articulation on the involved side. The dislocated vertebra and those above appear to be oblique on a lateral cervical spine film. The spinous processes of the vertebrae above the level of dislocation are displaced from the midline on AP roentgenograms.

HYPERFLEXION INJURIES

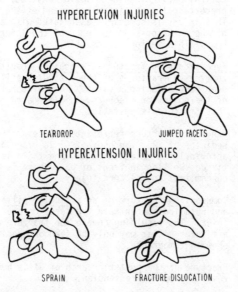

TEARDROP   JUMPED FACETS

HYPEREXTENSION INJURIES

SPRAIN   FRACTURE DISLOCATION

Figure 10.3.   The radiological picture of common cervical spine fractures.

d. Wedge compression fracture results in the decreased height of a vertebral body, especially anteriorly. Unless severe, this fracture is stable, but care should be taken that there is not an associated malignant tumor that has weakened the vertebral body, allowing it to fracture.

e. Tear drop fracture results from compression of the vertebral body. Lateral spine films demonstrate the tear drop as anteriorly displaced. A sagittal cleft passing through the vertebral body is seen on the AP projection. The displacement of the posterior edge of the vertebral body into the vertebral canal may result in an anterior spinal cord syndrome.

f. Clay-shoveler's fracture is the simple avulsion of a posterior spinous process.

2. Hyperextension Injuries

   a. <u>Hyperextension sprain</u> may result in extensive spinal
       cord damage with only subtle changes on the x-ray films.
       Lateral cervical spine films demonstrate widening of the
       prevertebral soft tissue space and of the disc space.
       This injury is sometimes associated with a chip fracture
       of the anterior-superior edge of the inferior vertebral
       body. This lesion is unstable.

   b. <u>Hyperextension fracture-dislocation</u> results in bilateral
       comminuted fractures of the articular pillars. This is
       seen best on oblique views. The vertebral body, freed
       of the posterior elements, is dislocated anteriorly.
       This fracture is unstable.

   c. <u>Hangman's fracture</u> represents bilateral fractures of the
       pedicles of C2. The body of C2 is often displaced
       anteriorly in relation to C3, and there is always soft
       tissue swelling in front of C2. There is usually no
       concomitant spinal cord injury.

   d. <u>Compression fracture of an articular pillar</u>. Extension
       and rotation concentrate the force on one apophyseal
       joint. The resulting compresion fracture of the
       articular pillar may only be seen on special x-ray views
       or with tomography.

   e. <u>Fracture of the posterior arch of C1</u> is benign and
       results from hyperextension.

3. Vertical Compression

   a. <u>Bursting fractures of the atlas</u>: Jefferson's fracture
       is the fracture of the anterior and posterior arches of
       the atlas and concomitant lateral displacement of the
       lateral masses. This lateral displacement can be
       appreciated on an AP x-ray film.

   b. <u>Burst fractures or comminuted fractures</u> of a lower
       cervical vertebral body can result in spinal cord injury
       by the displacement of bony fragments into the vertebral
       canal. AP views demonstrate a vertical fracture of the
       vertebral body. This fracture is stable.

D. Lumbar Spine Fractures

1. <u>Flexion wedge compression fractures</u> result from compression
    of the relatively soft cancellous bone of the lumbar
    vertebral body. Lateral lumbar spine films demonstrate a
    loss of height of the vertebral body, especially anteriorly,

or a discontinuity of the anterior cortical bone. When there is no clear history of trauma associated with this fracture, metastatic tumor or osteoporosis must be carefully searched for.

2. <u>Hyperflexion fractures</u> combine wedging of the vertebral body with disruption of the posterior elements. Because these fractures are unstable, the continuity of the posterior elements must be carefully scrutinized in all cases of wedge compression fractures. Widening of the distance between the pedicles, widening of the distance between adjacent posterior spinous processes, or separation of the posterior articulations indicate disruption of the posterior elements.

3. <u>Seat belt injuries</u> may be manifested as a distraction of the posterior elements or a horizontal fracture running through the posterior elements. These fractures are frequently associated with intra-abdominal trauma.

4. <u>Rotational fractures</u> result in a dislocation or fracture of the posterior elements. The vertebral body may suffer a horizontal fracture, or there may be a rupture of the disc bond. Transverse process fractures may be the only roentgenographic sign of these self-reducing fractures.

E. Care of the Patient with a Spinal Cord Injury

There is no specific therapy for already damaged nervous tissue. Treatment in the acute phase is aimed at decompression of the neural elements, stabilization of the spine, and avoidance of the systemic complications of hypoxia, hypotension, and infection. After the acute phase, therapy is aimed at rehabilitation.

1. Initial Management

    a. Establishment of an airway: Avoid neck movement if a cervical fracture is present. Use nasotracheal intubation or a tracheostomy if necessary.

    b. Evaluation and treatment of shock: Control external hemorrhage. Re-expand blood volume.

    c. Evaluation of other injuries.

    d. Neurological examination: Paraplegia or quadriplegia should be suspected in the unconscious patient who has a loss of deep tendon reflexes (spinal shock), no response to a painful stimulus below the level of the injury, or loss of intercostal respiration with abdominal breathing.

2. Care of the Spinal Injury

    a. Evaluation of spinal injury by multiple x-ray views, computed tomography, and myelography.

    b. Reduction of a fracture may be done under x-ray control using skeletal traction via a halo or cranial tongs. Occasionally the fracture must be exposed surgically to be reduced.

    c. The spine may be stabilized by a variety of methods, including bed rest, a cervical collar, a neck brace, cervical traction, a halo jacket, a corset, or a spica cast. Internal fixation can be accomplished with a spinal fusion or with inserted supports, such as Harrington rods.

    d. Surgical decompression may be necessary to remove a herniated disc fragment, hematoma, or bone spicule, especially if the patient's neurological status is deteriorating.

3. General Patient Care

    a. Respiratory status: Loss of intercostal muscle function may compromise respiration. Partial loss of phrenic function may also occur with high cervical lesions. Vigorous pulmonary toilet is required in patients with traumatic lesions of the cervical spinal cord.

    b. Loss of sympathetic tone occurs during the period of spinal shock. This may result in systemic hypotension (treated with intravascular fluid administration), poikilothermia or hypothermia, or hyperhidrosis (treated with an anticholinergic agent).

    c. Neurogenic bladder: Intermittent urinary catheterization is preferable to the insertion of an indwelling catheter. To reduce the risk of infection, give trimethoprim and sulfamethoxazole (2 tabs b.i.d.), methenamine mandelate (1 g q.i.d.) plus ascorbic acid (500 mg q.i.d.), or nitrofurantoin (50 mg q.i.d.).

    d. Skin care for the prevention of decubitus ulcers includes "log rolling" of the patient every 2 hours, the use of a sheepskin or alternating pressure mattress, padded booties, and good hygiene.

e. Adynamic ileus may persist for weeks. The patient
    should receive nothing by mouth and be maintained on
    intravenous fluids until bowel sounds return.
    Nasogastric drainage and a rectal tube for decompression
    are also worthwhile in the initial period after injury.
    A bisacodyl suppository given on alternate days will
    regulate the patient's bowel movements after the
    adynamic ileus subsides.

f. The incidence of thrombophlebitis can be reduced with
    elastic stockings and low-dose heparin (5,000 units q
    6-12 h subcutaneously).

g. Hypercalcuria from inactivity should be diluted with
    early hydration to avoid renal lithiasis.

h. Protein catabolism interferes with wound healing and
    resolution of infection. Parenteral hyperalimentation
    may be necessary.

i. High-dose steroid administration begun soon after injury
    may improve neurological recovery from spinal cord
    injury.

j. Peptic ulceration may develop secondary to stress and
    high dose steroids. This should be treated with
    antacids and cimetidine 300 mg i.v. q 8 h.

k. Spasticity can be treated medically with dantrolene (up
    to 100 mg q.i.d.), baclofen (up to 20 mg t.i.d.), or
    diazepam (up to 10 mg q.i.d.). Surgical treatment
    includes multiple rhizotomies, Bischoff's myelotomy, and
    the intrathecal injection of alcohol or phenol.

F. Diseases of the Spine

A loss of the normal trabeculated bone pattern in the vertebral
body is usually the first radiographic sign of a metastatic tumor to
the spine. The tumor may cause a compression fracture or collapse of
the vertebral body and eventually erodes through the bony cortex.
Characteristically, the disc space is preserved until very extensive
destruction has taken place. Metastatic tumor to the thoracic spine
can often be detected by the loss of a pedicle or pedicles as seen on
the AP x-ray view. Sclerosis can occur with metastatic prostatic
carcinoma and with breast carcinoma. Extensive tumor growth results
in epidural spinal cord compression and may necessitate surgical
decompression.

Unlike tumor, infection begins in the bony end plate adjoining
the intervertebral disc space. As the infection progresses, there is
a loss of height of the disc and destruction of the cortical bone at
the end plates of the adjacent vertebral bodies. The initial

manifestation of the infection is pain. The accumulation of pus under the posterior longitudinal ligament and in the epidural space may impinge on the nerve roots or the spinal cord to cause radiculopathy or myelopathy. Such infection is most commonly caused by Staphylococcus aureus. Pott's disease, tuberculosis of the spine, is a similar form of spinal osteomyelitis that results in kyphosis and epidural granulation tissue.

Ankylosing spondylitis, which presents as lumbar or interscapular pain, is characterized by progressive calcification of the spinal ligaments. Stiffness and limitation of motion insidiously spread to involve the entire spine with fusion of the costovertebral joints, limiting chest expansion. The calcified ligaments are responsible for the characteristic "bamboo" appearance seen on spinal roentgenograms. Extra-articular manifestations include iritis, aortic insufficiency, heart block, and ulcerative colitis.

Spondylolysis refers to a cleft in the pars interarticularis. This appears on the oblique x-ray film as a break in the neck of the Scottie dog. Spondylolisthesis refers to the displacement of one vertebral body on another. Spondylolysis and spondylolisthesis are most frequently combined at the lumbosacral junction. In this case, the L5 nerve roots may be compressed by the pseudarthrosis of the pars defect, causing radicular pain. Treatment for the radicular pain is surgical decompression; this is usually combined with posterolateral lumbar fusion.

Spondylosis (degenerative osteoarthritis of the spine) is a degenerative condition which may become symptomatic as pain, myelopathy, or radiculopathy. The degeneration is characterized by osteophyte formation along the margins of the vertebral end plates, and hypertrophy of the apophyseal joints. Bony spurs along the vertebral margins can be responsible for encroachment into the neural foramina (resulting in radiculopathy) or narrowing of the spinal canal (resulting in spinal cord or cauda equina impingement). Cervical spurs projecting anteriorly have been thought to be a cause of dysphagia, and lateral spurs have been said to be responsible for vertebral arterial insufficiency. Both of these manifestations are rare.

Rheumatoid arthritis is characterized by intra-articular and joint capsule inflammation. Three manifestations may develop in the cervical spine: (1) loosening of the atlantoaxial ligaments with C1-C2 subluxation, (2) alterations in the ligaments of the articular facets which lead to anterior dislocation of one vertebral body on another, and (3) upward displacement of the dens into the foramen magnum.

Achondroplasia, the most common form of dwarfism, comes to the attention of the neurosurgeon because of stenosis of the spinal canal and narrowing of the intervertebral foramina. Increased kyphosis caused by wedging of the vertebrae at the thoracolumbar junction make this area particularly vulnerable to spinal cord compression. Shortening of the dens poses the threat of C1-C2 subluxation.

REFERENCES

Braakman R, Penning L: Injuries of the Cervical Spine. Amsterdam, Excerpta Medica, 1971.

Dolan KD: Radiological determination of cervical spine fracture and stability. Clin Neurosurg 27:368-384, 1980.

Gehweiler JA, Osborne RL, Becker RF: The Radiology of Vertebral Trauma. Philadelphia, WB Saunders, 1980.

Perrin RG, Livingston KE: Neurological treatment of pathological fracture-dislocation of the spine. J Neurosurg 52:330-334, 1980.

Chapter 11

The Spinal Cord

Fully evolved spinal cord lesions are easily identified. The challenge lies in the early recognition of the vague warning symptoms which precede a permanent devastating spinal cord impairment.

A. Functional Anatomy of the Spinal Cord (Fig. 11.1)

1. The spinal cord ordinarily terminates in a leash of nerves, the cauda equina, at the level of the L1 vertebra. These nerve roots supply the lower extremities, bowel, and bladder. In the usual circumstance, vertebral lesions below the L1 vertebra cannot cause spinal cord damage but only nerve root compression.

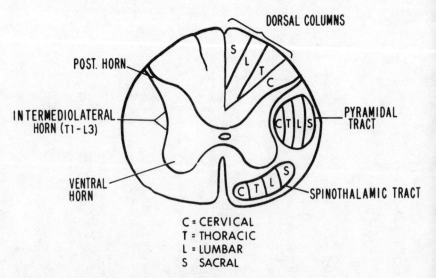

Figure 11.1. Spinal cord anatomy.

2. Lower motor neurons (LMNs), whose axons make up the motor
nerves, reside in the ipsilateral ventral horn of the spinal
cord. Lower motor neuron lesions produce muscular wasting
which may be identified by the examiner before the patient
notices significant weakness. Fasciculations signify motor
neuron damage at or near the cell bodies within the spinal
cord. When lower motor neurons are injured, the muscles they
supply become weak and hypotonic.

3. Upper motor neurons, whose axons end on the contralateral
LMNs, originate in the cerebral cortex. The majority of
these axons travel through the pyramidal tract in the
posterolateral portion of the spinal cord where they maintain
topographical order with the fibers subserving the leg
lateral to those regulating the arm. Patients note upper
motor neuron lesions as minor incoordination before weakness
becomes manifest on examination. Physical examination may
reveal (below the level of the lesion) brisk deep tendon
reflexes, increased muscle tone, extensor plantar (Babinski)
responses, and difficulty performing rapid alternating
motions following spinal shock.

4. Fibers mediating pain and temperature sensation cross to the
opposite side of the spinal cord within three spinal segments
of their entry. They travel up the contralateral side of the
cord in the lateral spinothalamic tract.

5. Position sensation is mediated through the dorsal columns.
These fibers are arranged in a centrifugal pattern with the
fibers from the upper extremity located lateral to those from
the lower extremity. Patients with lesions of the dorsal
column complain of tingling, paresthesias, or numbness. The
anatomical localization of vibratory sensation remains
uncertain.

6. Joint position sensation that does not reach the level of
consciousness travels in the spinocerebellar tracts. These
tracts are most conspicuously affected in the spinocerebellar
degenerations, such as Friedreich's ataxia.

7. Sympathetic fibers travel caudally within the cord to T1-L3
and synapse in the intermediate horn.

8. The vascular supply of the anterior two-thirds of the spinal
cord is derived from radicals of the anterior spinal artery.
This artery is fed by six to eight branches from the
radicular arteries at irregular intervals along the cord.
The most prominent feeding vessel is the artery of
Adamkiewicz which originates most frequently from a left
radicular artery between T9 and L2. Occlusion of the
anterior spinal artery can result from small emboli,

dissection of the aorta, thrombosis of the distal aorta, or atherosclerotic disease. The posterior one-third of the spinal cord derives its blood supply from paired posterior spinal arteries.

B. Spinal Cord Lesions

   1. Traumatic lesions of the spinal cord manifest certain characteristics depending on the anatomy of the lesion (Fig. 11.2).

      a. Anterior cord syndrome is frequently vascular in origin resulting from compression or occlusion of the anterior spinal artery or occlusion of a major radicular artery as seen with a dissecting aortic aneurysm. Its characteristics are:

         i. Complete paralysis below the level of injury.

         ii. Hypalgesia and hypesthesia below the level of injury.

         iii. Preservation of position and vibratory sensation.

SYNDROMES

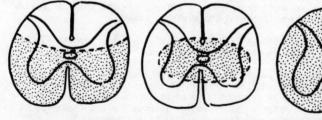

ANT. CORD SYNDROME   CENTRAL CORD   BROWN-SEQUARD

Figure 11.2. Area of spinal cord damaged in three classic spinal cord syndromes.

b. Central cord syndrome is most commonly seen after trauma in a patient with pre-existing cervical spinal stenosis. Its characteristics are:

   i. Greater loss of motor power in the upper extremities than in the lower extremities.

   ii. Variable degree of sensory loss.

   iii. Recovery follows the specific pattern of lower extremities recovering first, the arms next, and the hands last.

   iv. Urinary retention occurs in more severe cases.

c. The Brown-Séquard syndrome results from a hemisection of the spinal cord. Its characteristics are:

   i. Ipsilateral spastic paralysis below the level of the lesion.

   ii. Ipsilateral reduction in position and vibratory sensation below the level of the lesion.

   iii. Contralateral loss of pain and temperature sensation beginning one or two dermatomes below the level of the lesion.

   iv. A radicular band of anesthesia and flaccid paralysis on the ipsilateral side at the level of the lesion.

d. Spinal shock follows acute severe spinal cord injury and lasts from days to weeks. Its characteristics are:

   i. Loss of reflex function in all segments of the spinal cord below the level of the lesion.

   ii. Atonic dysfunction of the bladder.

2. Compressive or expanding lesions of the spinal cord follow certain patterns.

a. Extrinsic Cord Compression Syndrome

   i. Pain at the level of the lesion is frequently exacerbated by the Valsalva maneuver or percussion of the vertebrae at the involved level.

   ii. Signs of pyramidal tract damage are the most striking initial findings.

      iii. Difficulty initiating micturition may then be
            followed by urinary retention.

      iv. Sensory loss may be radicular at the level of
            the lesion or may occur as an ascending sensory
            level.

      v. Lhermitte's sign, in which neck flexion produces
            electrical paresthesias radiating down the spine
            and into the limbs, may be a symptom of cervical
            spinal cord compression or of an intrinsic spinal
            cord lesion in the cervical area.

   b. Intrinsic Lesions

      i. Pain and temperature fibers which decussate at the
            level of the lesion are impaired, yielding a band
            of dissociated sensory loss (pain sensation lost,
            position sensation retained).

      ii. Pain tends to be burning, poorly localized, and
            worse at night.

      iii. Invasion of gray matter results in segmental loss
            of deep tendon reflexes, muscle wasting, weakness,
            fasciculations, and, in the cervical region,
            Horner's syndrome.

      iv. Long tracts are involved late in the disease
            processes, and the medial portions mediating
            function of the upper extremity are more severely
            affected than the laterally placed fibers
            subserving leg, bowel, and bladder functions
            (sacral sparing).

C. Spinal Cord Tumors

   1. Spinal cord tumors are classified by the compartment in which
      they appear -- intramedullary, intradural extramedullary, and
      extradural. A lesion in each compartment has a
      characteristic myelographic picture (Fig. 11.3).

   2. Myelography (Fig. 11.3) is performed by filling the
      subarachnoid space with a radiopaque contrast agent.
      Intramedullary tumors demonstrate a widening of the spinal
      cord which displaces the contrast laterally. Intradural
      extramedullary tumors displace the spinal cord, enlarging the
      subarachnoid space above and below the tumor. This enlarged
      space appears as a cap of contrast above and below the
      lesion. Extradural lesions displace both the contrast
      material and the spinal cord.

MYELOGRAPHIC APPEARANCE OF SPINAL TUMORS

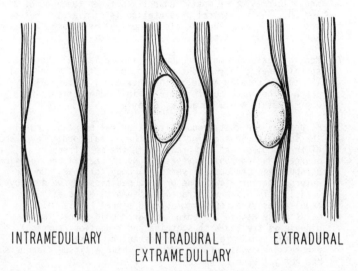

INTRAMEDULLARY   INTRADURAL   EXTRADURAL
                      EXTRAMEDULLARY

Figure 11.3.   The myelographic medium is represented by the lined
areas which outline the spinal cord (white central zone).

3.   Astrocytomas of all grades occur most frequently in the
     cervical spinal cord. These tumors frequently occur in
     childhood and may be cystic. Occasionally the tumor can be
     surgically extirpated from the cord.

4.   Ependymomas occur most often in males and are frequently
     found in the low cervical spinal cord where there is a high
     incidence of an associated syrinx. A second group of
     ependymomas involves the filum terminale in the lumbar canal.

5.   Schwannomas occur most often in the extramedullary intradural
     space in patients 30-60 years of age. They usually present
     with radicular pain or spinal cord compression. Plain x-ray
     films may demonstrate an enlarged neural foramen. They are
     sometimes multiple and may be associated with

von Recklinghausen's disease. Occasionally, a schwannoma assumes a dumbbell shape through the neural foramen, coming to clinical attention as an intrathoracic or intra-abdominal mass.

6. Neurofibromas occur most frequently between the ages of 30 and 50. Their clinical presentation is similar to that of schwannomas, and they are also sometimes associated with von Recklinghausen's disease.

7. Meningiomas occur most frequently in the lateral thoracic spinal canal. They almost never occur in the lumbar canal. The tumors usually arise in the intradural extramedullary space. They occur preferentially in female patients at approximately a 9:1 female:male ratio.

8. Metastases are most frequently extradural but can occur in the subarachnoid space or within the spinal cord. Carcinoma of the lung, breast, or prostate is the most frequent primary source. Radiographic investigations may reveal bony erosion, osteoblastic changes, or vertebral body collapse. On the anteroposterior views, one or more pedicles may be destroyed. Occasionally primary intracranial tumors, especially medulloblastomas, ependymomas, and pineal tumors will metastasize within the spinal subarachnoid space. Metastatic disease is treated with steroids and radiation; surgical decompression is reserved for refractory or rapidly progressing cases, or for cases in which a tissue diagnosis has not yet been established.

9. Chordomas are rare tumors which originate from remnants of the notochord. Of spinal chordomas, 80% are sacrococcygeal in location.

10. Lipomas can be intra- or extradural. The intradural lipomas are usually within and dorsal to the lumbosacral portion of the spinal cord. Such a lipoma can occur as a part of a spinal dysplasia (lipomeningocele) where it is associated with tethering of the spinal cord and involvement of the cauda equina by the lipoma.

11. Cysts

    a. Epidermoids may begin de novo or result from bits of skin implanted in the lumbar canal at the time of lumbar puncture.

Table 11.1.
Most Common Spinal Tumors

	Adult	Child
Intramedullary	Ependymoma Astrocytoma Hemangioblastoma	Astrocytoma Epidermoid/dermoid Ependymoma

Intradural,
extramedullary
	Neurofibroma
	Schwannoma
	Meningioma
	Metastases from
	  intracranial tumor
	Ependymoma of filum
	  terminale
		Lipoma
		Angioma
		Neurofibroma

Extradural	Metastasis Myeloma Lymphoma Chordoma Sarcoma	Neuroblastoma Lymphoma Sarcoma

      b. Dermoid cysts occur most commonly in the conus
medullaris. Such a dermoid cyst may be attached to the
skin via a dermal sinus tract that extends the
lower lumbar spine or sacrum.

      c. Neurenteric cysts, lined by mucus-secreting epithelium,
and arachnoid cysts, derived from arachnoidal
diverticula, are other types of cysts that may occur in
the spinal canal.

   12. <u>Hemangioblastomas</u> are highly vascular tumors which occur as
isolated entities or in association with other manifestations
of Lindau's disease. If a cleavage plane can be established,
these tumors may be extirpated from the cord.

D. Other Spinal Disorders

    1. <u>Syringomyelia</u> refers to a cavitation of the spinal cord
originating in the gray matter. A syrinx may occur in
association with a spinal cord tumor but most frequently
occurs alone or in association with a congenital malformation
at the craniocervical junction, such as the Arnold-Chiari
malformation. Patients with syringomyelia present with a
dissociated loss of pain sensation and progressive wasting of
the small muscles of the hands. Two forms of treatment
involve decompressing the fourth ventricle (when there is an

associated Arnold-Chiari malformation) or shunting the cyst
into the subarachnoid space.

2. Vascular malformations, which usually lie on the dorsal
    surface or deep within the spinal cord, come to clinical
    attention because of a neurological deficit or subarachnoid
    hemorrhage.

3. Spontaneous epidural hematomas, which are most frequently
    located in the thoracic region, are seen in association with
    anticoagulant therapy, blood dyscrasias, coagulopathies, or
    epidural vascular malformations. The hematoma is usually
    heralded by pain prior to the ensuing neurological deficit.

4. Epidural and subdural abscesses are usually caused by a
    Staphylococcus infection but may be due to any organism.
    They are discussed in association with other infectious
    diseases (see Chapter 13).

5. Multiple sclerosis, a demyelinating disease which may cause a
    variety of neurological symptoms, can present as an acute or
    subacute transverse spinal cord lesion (transverse myelitis)
    that tends to improve with time.

6. Amyotrophic lateral sclerosis is a progressive degenerative
    disease involving both upper and lower motor neurons. Either
    of these two components may be predominant. Involvement of
    the lower cranial nerves carries a particularly poor
    prognosis.

7. Spinocerebellar degenerations are a set of familial diseases
    which cause progressive dysfunction of the spinal cord,
    cerebellum, and basal ganglia.

8. Subacute combined degeneration (B12 deficiency) manifests
    as a dysfunction of the dorsal columns and pyramidal tracts.
    The patient presents with fine tingling paresthesias. In
    advanced cases, psychosis may also be present.

9. Radiation myelopathy is a rapidly progressive transverse loss
    of spinal cord function which occurs 6-18 months following
    radiation therapy of the spine. This condition must be
    differentiated from cord compression by the tumor that was
    originally treated with radiotherapy.

REFERENCES

Black P: Spinal   metastasis: current   status   and   recommended
guidelines for management. Neurosurgery 5:726-746, 1979.

Malis LI: Microsurgery for spinal cord arteriovenous malformations.
Clin Neurosurg 26:543-555, 1979.

Schneider RC, Crosby EC, Russon RH, et al: Traumatic spinal cord
syndromes and their management. Clin Neurosurg 20:424-492, 1973.

Stein BM: Surgery of intramedullary spinal cord tumors.   Clin
Neurosurg 26:529-542, 1979.

Yasouka S, Okazakoui H, Duabe JR, et al: Foramen magnum tumors:
analysis of 57 cases of benign extramedullary tumors.   J
Neurosurg 49:828-838, 1978.

Chapter 12

Peripheral and Cranial Nerves

In order to make the diagnosis of a peripheral nerve lesion, the normal pattern of sensory and motor composition of peripheral nerves and nerve roots must be appreciated (Fig. 12.1). The physician can then compare the patient's symptoms and physical findings with the known anatomy of the peripheral nerves in order to determine the locus of the lesion.

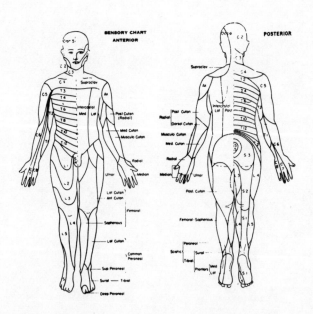

Figure 12.1. Sensory distribution of dermatomes and major nerves. (Reprinted from Haymaker W, Woodhall B: _Peripheral Nerve Injuries: Principles of Diagnosis_, ed 2. Philadelphia, W. B. Saunders Co., 1953.)

A. The Upper Extremity

   1. Nerve Roots

      Injury to the innervation of the upper extremity can occur
      at the level of the nerve roots, the brachial plexus, or
      along the peripheral nerves. The arm is innervated by the
      fifth cervical through first thoracic nerve roots. The main
      distribution of each nerve root is outlined in Table 12.1.
      Although most muscles are innervated by multiple roots, Table
      12.1 notes their predominant innervation. Roots are affected
      by:

      a. Compression from herniated disc, arthritic ridge
          (spondylosis), vertebral fracture, or tumor.

      b. Traumatic avulsion

   2. Herniated Discs (Fig. 12.2)

      a. The intervertebral disc is composed of a soft fibrous
          center, the nucleus pulposus, surrounded by a tough
          covering, the annulus fibrosus. A herniated ("slipped")
          disc occurs when a portion of the nucleus pulposus
          ruptures through a rent in the annulus fibrosus.

          It is thought that the partially extruded fragment of
          nucleus pulposus causes localized pain by distorting the
          pain-sensitive annulus fibrosus and posterior
          longitudinal ligament. The patient with a partially
          extruded cervical disc often has dull aching pain which
          radiates into the shoulder, medial scapula, and anterior
          upper thorax. A patient with partial lumbar disc
          extrusion often presents with similar pain in the low
          back radiating into the hip. When the fragment
          completely extrudes, new symptoms occur, resulting from
          compression of a nerve root within the spinal canal.

      b. Acute lateral cervical disc herniation presents as pain
          which initially may be localized to the neck, medial
          scapula, and upper chest. Radicular symptoms and signs
          of nerve root compression follow. These include pain
          radiating into the arm, weakness, fasciculations, loss
          of sensation, and loss of reflexes in a specific
          distribution (see Table 12.1). The most common level
          of cervical disc herniation is the C6 disc (between the
          C6 and C7 vertebrae).

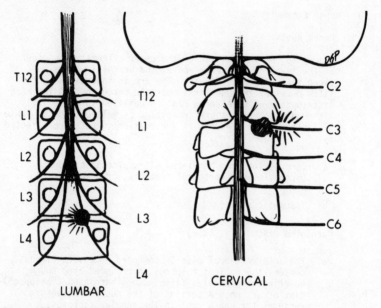

LUMBAR   CERVICAL

Figure 12.2. Herniated lumbar and cervical discs. Note that the herniated cervical disc affects the nerve root exiting at the level of the herniation whereas the herniated lumbar disc compresses the nerve root exiting at the next lower level.

    c. Physical examination also reveals that:

       i. Pain is exacerbated by:

         a) Pressing on the vertex of the head with the head tilted toward the painful side (Spurling's maneuver).

         b) Extending the patient's neck.

         c) Rotating the neck away from the side of the lesion.

         d) Percussing the spinous processes of the involved vertebrae.

       ii. The pain may be relieved by pulling the head in a straight line with the spinal axis

      iii. If the disc protrudes centrally, signs of spinal cord compression can be demonstrated.

Table 12.1.
Deficit Resulting from Cervical Nerve Root Injury

	Disc: C4 Nerve Root: C5	Disc: C5 Nerve Root: C6	Disc: C6 Nerve Root: C7	Disc: C7 Nerve Root: C8
Sensory loss	Shoulder and lateral arm	Radial aspect of forearm, thumb, and index finger	Posterior arm, posterior forearm, index and long fingers	Medial forearm and ulnar two fingers
Motor weakness	Shoulder abductors (supraspinatus and deltoid) Shoulder external rotators (infraspinatus) Internal rotators of shoulder (sub-scapularis, teres minor) Scapular adductors (rhomboids)	Elbow flexors (biceps, brachialis, brachioradialis) Forearm supinators (supinator; biceps) Forearm pronators (pronator teres, pronator quadratus)	Wrist extensors (extensor carpi radialis longus and brevis, extensor carpi ulnaris) Elbow extensors (triceps) Shoulder adductors (latissimus dorsi, pectoralis major)	Finger flexors (flexor digitorum profundus, flexor digitorum sublimis) Ulnar deviator of the hand (flexor carpi ulnaris)
Changes in deep tendon reflexes	Biceps reflex may be mildly diminished	Biceps and radial reflexes diminished or absent	Triceps reflex diminished or absent	Finger flexor reflex diminished or absent

    d. Unless the patient has weakness or significant myelo-
pathy, a trial of bed rest, longitudinal cervical
traction, muscle relaxants, anti-inflammatory agents,
and/or mild analgesics is indicated. Plain x-ray films
of the cervical spine are obtained to rule out other
causes of neck and arm pain. If conservative therapy
fails, the diagnosis may be confirmed by myelography,
and the extruded disc fragment may be removed by a
posterior partial hemilaminectomy or via an anterior
approach through the intervertebral disc.

3. Cervical Spondylosis

    a. Osteoarthritis also may encroach on a nerve root in the
neural foramen, causing a painful radiculopathy. This
occurs most frequently at the C5-6 interspace but may
involve other or multiple levels of the cervical spine.
In general, the symptoms and signs of cervical
osteoarthritis (cervical spondylosis) causing
radiculopathy are similar to those of cervical disc
herniation. However, the evolution of symptoms is
insidious when compared with those of an acute disc
herniation. Also, the pain and paresthesias of
spondylosis may be worse in the morning when the patient
first awakens. When multiple levels of spondylotic
radiculopathy are combined with myelopathy, the clinical
picture may mimic amyotrophic lateral sclerosis.

    b. The encroachment of spondylotic ridges into the neural
foramen is best seen in oblique roentgenograms of the
cervical spine. Myelography demonstrates concomitant
nerve root compression. If conservative therapy
(similar to that used for cervical disc herniation)
fails to relieve the patient's pain, surgical
decompression is indicated, either through an anterior
or a posterior approach.

4. Fractures of the Spine

These cause radicular symptoms by contusing or lacerating one
or more nerve roots.

5. Tumors

    a. Neurofibromas and schwannomas can occur anywhere along
the course of a peripheral nerve. A schwannoma almost
always originates from a single sensory fascicle. A
neurofibroma involves the entire nerve, incorporating
all the fascicles of the nerve within its mass. Thus a
schwannoma can frequently be resected leaving the
majority of the nerve intact, whereas the removal of a
neurofibroma necessitates sacrificing the nerve.

b. Peripheral tumors may present as a progressive mononeuropathy or as a painful, tender mass. Tumors within the cervical and thoracic spine cause spinal cord compression. Tumors occurring high in the lumbar canal compress the conus, causing urinary retention, perirectal pain, and saddle numbness. The cauda equina may be compressed by a schwannoma, neurofibroma, ependymoma, lipoma, or epidermoid tumor.

c. Metastatic tumors usually cause radiculopathy by epidural compression of one or more spinal nerve roots. Lower extremity radiculopathies are a frequent presentation of meningeal carcinomatosis.

d. Myelography is the definitive test for tumors within the spinal canal.

6. Brachial Plexus Lesions

a. Brachial plexus injuries usually result from a stretch of the plexus during trauma or, less frequently, from a direct penetrating injury. In patients with direct penetration, damage to the lung, subclavian/axillary artery, or subclavian/axillary vein must be considered.

i. Injury to the brachial plexus may take place at the level of the nerve roots, above the clavicle, or below the clavicle (see Table 12.2). Actual avulsion of one or more nerve roots from the spinal cord can be anticipated when physical examination reveals dysfunction of the:

a) Long thoracic nerve (winging of the scapula),

b) Dorsal scapular nerve (weakness of the rhomboids),

c) Phrenic nerve (paralysis and elevation of the ipsilateral diaphragm), or

d) Sympathetic nerves (Horner's syndrome).

ii. Nerve root avulsions have a hopeless prognosis, whereas infraclavicular lesions of the plexus may have an excellent prognosis for return of function. Supraclavicular lesions not involving the nerve roots may be helped on occasion, and usually warrant surgical exploration.

iii. Signs of brachial plexus dysfunction progressing
after the injury may result from an expanding
arterial aneurysm or exuberant callus formation
around a clavicular fracture.

b. Thoracic outlet syndrome may present as a position-
dependent occlusion of the subclavian artery or vein, as
Raynaud's phenomenon, or (most often) as a lower
brachial plexus syndrome. The neurological syndrome is
manifested as aching pain in the axilla and along the
ulnar border of the forearm. As the syndrome
progresses, weakness occurs in the small muscles of the
hand. A supraclavicular bruit is frequently heard.

c. Brachial neuritis (Parsonage-Turner syndrome) refers to
idiopathic focal upper extremity weakness and atrophy.
The weakness may follow an immunization or viral
illness. It is heralded by severe aching neck and
shoulder pain and may be accompanied by paresthesias or
spotty, nondermatomal sensory loss. The weakness and
atrophy are usually confined to the large proximal
muscles.

7. Peripheral Nerve Entrapment

a. The suprascapular nerve may become entrapped in the
scapular notch. The patient complains of deep aching
pain over the shoulder which is exacerbated by forward
rotation of the shoulder. Weakness may be detected in
initiating abduction (supraspinatus) and in externally
rotating the shoulder (infraspinatus).

b. The axillary nerve which innervates the deltoid and
teres minor and mediates sensation over the deltoid may
be injured as a result of a humeral fracture, shoulder
dislocation, or deep intramuscular injection. Rarely,
the axillary nerve can be entrapped as it passes through
the quadrilateral space.

c. The median nerve is most frequently entrapped at the
wrist or in the forearm (see Table 12.3).

i. Carpal tunnel syndrome occurs when the median nerve
is compressed as it passes under the flexor
retinaculum (within the carpal tunnel) in the wrist
and palm. Patients complain of paresthesias in the
sensory distribution of the median nerve which are
most severe at night. In more advanced cases, the
patient will have weakness of abduction and
opposition of the thumb and wasting of the lateral
thenar eminence. Tinel's sign can be elicited over
the median nerve at the wrist, and hyperflexion of

Table 12.2.
The Brachial Plexus

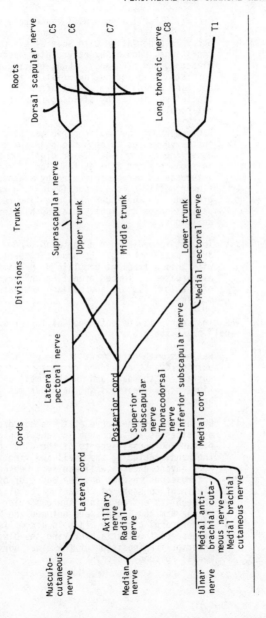

the wrist for 1 minute will exacerbate the pain (Phalen's sign). The carpal tunnel syndrome can occur in association with several systemic conditions, such as hypothyroidism, acromegaly, diabetes, and pregnancy. Conservative therapy consists of splinting the wrist in the neutral position during sleep. Most often the syndrome is treated surgically by dividing the flexor retinaculum.

ii.   Entrapment of the median nerve may also occur as the nerve passes through the pronator teres and under the edge of the flexor digitorum sublimis. This can present as a dysfunction of the anterior interosseous nerve manifested by weakness of the flexor pollicis longus and flexor digitorum profundus of the index and long fingers. The patient notes difficulty flexing his terminal phalanges.

iii.   The entire median nerve may also become entrapped as it passes through the pronator teres. Patients with this entrapment complain of proximal arm pain exacerbated by forced pronation and have weakness of the long flexors and median innervated intrinsic muscles.

d. The ulnar nerve may be entrapped at the wrist (Guyon's canal) or at the elbow.

i.   Patients with entrapment at the wrist complain of burning dysesthesias and numbness over the ulnar surface of the palm and in the small and ring fingers, and weakness in the ulnar muscles of the hand.

ii.   Entrapment of the nerve at the elbow presents as dysesthesias and a change in sensation over the palmar and dorsal aspects of the ulnar portion of the hand, including the small and ring fingers. More advanced cases will manifest weakness of the interosseous muscles and the adductor of the thumb. Treatment consists of releasing the ulnar nerve between its entrance into the posterior compartment of the arm and its passage between the heads of the flexor carpi ulnaris. This is accomplished by a release of the fascia overlying the ulnar nerve, an anterior transposition of the ulnar nerve, or a medial epicondylectomy.

Table 12.3.
Innervation of Arm

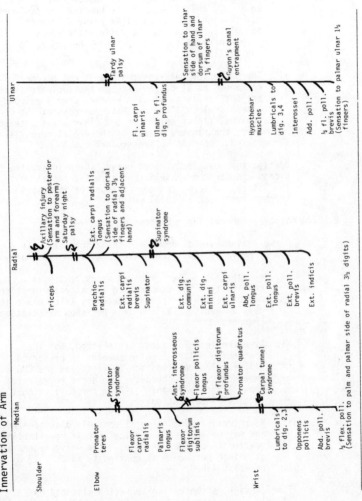

e. The radial nerve is prone to be injured in three separate locations.

    i. Injury in the axilla or as the nerve spirals around the humerus is the result of sudden trauma (e.g., an injury that fractures the humerus) or prolonged compression ("Saturday night palsy," "crutch palsy"). The two can be differentiated by involvement of the triceps when the injury is in the axilla.

    ii. The posterior interosseous branch can become entrapped as it passes through the supinator. The patient complains of pain at the lateral epicondyle ("tennis elbow") and may have weakness of the proximal finger extensors and ulnar wrist extensor. Since the sensory branch of the radial nerve is spared, there is no sensory deficit.

f. Rarely, the musculocutaneous nerve, which innervates the biceps and coracobrachialis and supplies sensation to the lateral forearm, can be entrapped as it passes through the coracobrachial muscle.

8. Traumatic Peripheral Nerve Lesions

a. Nerve lesions are graded as to their severity. In about 60% of nerve lesions, the nerve remains in continuity.

    i. Neurapraxia: The nerve and axons remain in continuity. The sensory and sympathetic functions may be partially spared. Recovery takes place in days or weeks. The EMG does not show denervation changes.

    ii. Axonotmesis: The axons are severed, but the continuity of the Schwann sheaths is preserved. All neurological function is lost, and the EMG will show denervation changes. The nerve regenerates at about 1 inch per month (1-2 mm per day) without surgical intervention.

    iii. Neurotmesis: The nerve is entirely disorganized and may be severed. Surgical repair re-establishes continuity of the fascicles. The nerve regenerates at 1 inch per month if continuity is re-established.

b. Tinel's sign, a shock-like sensation elicited by lightly percussing the nerve, is indicative of regenerating sensory fibers. Tinel's sign can always be elicited at the site of injury, but if it is present further down the nerve, it indicates advancing small sensory fibers. Unfortunately, there is no guarantee that larger motor fibers will follow. Since small sympathetic fibers regenerate quickest, the return of sweating is a hopeful sign.

c. Causalgia is a syndrome characterized by severe burning pain following a nerve injury. It may spread beyond the distribution of the involved nerve or nerves, and it is usually aggravated by physical and emotional stimuli. It may be accompanied by excessive sweating and trophic changes distal to the injury. The pain is characteristically eased by local application of water or by sympathetic blockade. The syndrome usually occurs in conjunction with a partial nerve injury, especially one caused by a high-velocity bullet.

d. The shoulder-hand syndrome (one form of reflex sympathetic dystrophy) refers to a painful and progressive limitation of the movement of a shoulder associated with swelling, stiffness, and discoloration of the ipsilateral hand. Without treatment, when the acute phase resolves in 3-6 months, the patient may be left with flexion contractures and trophic changes in the hand. This condition may occur following other conditions that cause pain in, or limit the movement of, the shoulder and arm, such as shoulder trauma, stroke, or myocardial infarction. It should be treated early, with techniques to reduce pain (e.g., sympathetic or peripheral nerve blocks) and improve the range of shoulder motion.

B. The Lower Extremity

The lumbar and sacral nerve roots, which innervate the lower extremities, bowel, and bladder, originate from the termination of the spinal cord between T10 and L1. These nerves then traverse the lower spinal canal before exiting at their respective neural foramina. Therefore, lesions of the lumbar canal can cause radiculopathies but not a myelopathy.

1. Lumbar Disc Herniation

a. A herniated lumbar disc may entrap any nerve root passing through the neural canal at the level of the herniation. Most often the nerve root exiting through the neural foramen one segment below the herniated disc is affected, i.e., an L4 disc herniation presents with an L5 radiculopathy. Most lumbar disc herniations involve the L4 or L5 disc (L5 or S1 nerve root). The patients usually give a history of intermittent back pain which then becomes accompanied by unilateral pain

in the distribution of the sciatic nerve (sciatica).
The pain is exacerbated by physical activity, prolonged
sitting, and the Valsalva maneuver.

b. Physical examination may reveal that the paravertebral
muscles are stiff on palpation. Low back movement is
restricted, and lumbar scoliosis may be present.

   i. Root entrapment is suspected when the radicular
   pain is exacerbated by one of several maneuvers:

      a) Flexing the hip while maintaining the knee in
      extension (Laseque's sign). In contrast,
      simultaneous hip and knee flexion do not
      stretch the sciatic nerve and its component
      nerve roots and do not exacerbate the pain.
      If straight leg raising of the nonpainful leg
      causes pain in the involved leg (Fajersztajn's
      sign), a free fragment of extruded disc
      material may be present at the axilla of the
      nerve root.

      b) Pulling the tibial nerve forward in the
      popliteal fossa with the hip and knee flexed
      (popliteal compression test).

      c) Pressing on the sciatic nerve at the sciatic
      notch.

      d) Extending the hip which may exacerbate pain
      resulting from a L4 root entrapment (femoral
      stretch sign).

   ii. Hip pain on internal or external rotation of the
   hip or with simultaneous hip and knee flexion is
   indicative of local hip disease.

   iii. Radicular signs include fasciculations, weakness,
   loss of sensation, and reflex changes in a specific
   distribution (see Table 12.4).

c. Patients with a suspected disc herniation who do not
have associated weakness or bowel or bladder dysfunction
can be treated with bed rest and analgesics. Plain
x-ray films of the lumbosacral spine are obtained to
rule out other causes of back and leg pain (e.g., tumor,
spondylolisthesis). If the pain does not subside in 2
weeks, the diagnosis of a herniated disc can be
confirmed by myelography or spinal CT scan. The
herniated disc may be removed through a partial
hemilaminectomy.

Table 12.4.
Deficit Resulting from Lumbosacral Nerve Root Lesion

	Root				
	L2	L3	L4	L5	S1	S2-3
Distribution of sensory loss	Anterosuperior thigh	Anterior thigh	Anterior thigh and medial leg to malleolus	Lateral leg and dorsum of the foot to large toe	Lateral leg and foot to small toe	Buttocks and genitals
Motor weakness	Hip flexion, hip adduction	Hip adduction, knee extension	Knee extension, foot inversion	Foot and toe extension	Foot flexion and rarely foot eversion	Toe flexion; paralysis of small muscles of foot resulting in (clawing of toes)
Alterations in reflexes		Adductor reflex diminished or absent	Knee jerk diminished or absent		Ankle jerk diminished or absent	Parasympathetic bladder reflexes and penile erection

2. Lumbar Spondylosis

    Osteoarthritis may present clinically as back pain or back
    pain and radiculopathy. The pain is aching in nature and is
    exacerbated by prolonged standing and walking. More than one
    nerve root may be involved. The diagnosis of lumbar
    spondylosis is made by plain x-ray films. The degree of
    spinal stenosis or nerve root compression is assessed by
    myelography or spinal CT scan.

3. Neurogenic Claudication

    Neurogenic claudication is associated with lumbar spinal
    stenosis. The patient experiences aching pain, paresthesias,
    and numbness in the legs associated with walking, prolonged
    standing, or any activity in which the lumbar spine is held
    in extension. The discomfort is relieved by rest and flexion
    of the lumbar spine. Unlike ischemic claudication, the
    discomfort associated with neurogenic claudication may
    develop while the patient is standing quietly.

4. Peripheral Nerve Entrapment

    a. Entrapment of the lateral femoral cutaneous nerve at the
        inguinal ligament results in painful paresthesias and
        numbness of the anterolateral aspect of the thigh. The
        discomfort is exacerbated by standing or walking.

    b. The obturator nerve, which carries sensation from the
        medial thigh and supplies the adductors of the thigh,
        can be involved by pelvic neoplasms, compressed during
        pregnancy, or entrapped in the obturator canal by an
        obturator hernia or osteitis pubis.

    c. The femoral nerve supplies motor fibers to the knee
        extensors (quadriceps) and hip flexors. It carries
        sensation to the anterior thigh and medial leg down to
        the medial malleolus. Injury to the nerve is associated
        with a loss of the knee jerk. Infarction of the nerve,
        which is not infrequent in the patient with diabetes
        mellitus, is associated with burning pain. The nerve
        may be damaged as it passes along the psoas muscle by a
        psoas abscess or retroperitoneal hematoma, or it may be
        entrapped at the level of the inguinal ligament by a
        femoral hernia or a femoral artery aneurysm. Rarely,
        the entrapment of the nerve at the knee (saphenous
        nerve) may result in medial leg pain.

    d. The sciatic nerve innervates the flexors of the knee and
        all of the muscles of the calf. It supplies sensation
        to the entire calf except for its medial aspect. The
        nerve is composed of two divisions, the common peroneal

Table 12.5.
Innervation of Leg

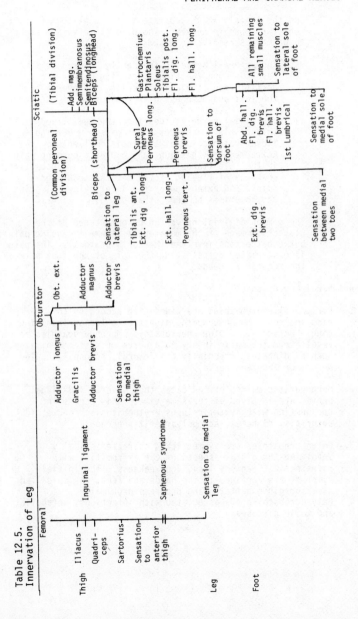

and the tibial, which separate in the popliteal fossa to form two separate nerves. The peroneal division seems to be more sensitive to trauma.

    i. The peroneal nerve is frequently injured as it passes around the fibula, causing weakness of dorsiflexion (tibialis anterior) and eversion of the foot and numbness over the dorsum of the foot.

   ii. The tibial nerve divides into the medial and lateral plantar nerves as it passes under the flexor retinaculum at the medial malleolus. Entrapment at this juncture causes a burning pain in the sole (tarsal tunnel syndrome). Concomitant weakness of flexion of the metatarsophalangeal joints and extension of the interphalangeal joints can sometimes be demonstrated.

  e. The common digital nerve can be compressed on the plantar surface of the metatarsal ligament causing pain between the toes involved (Morton's neuroma). The pain is exacerbated by palpating the sole of the foot between the metatarsal heads.

C. Peripheral Neuropathies

  1. Peripheral neuropathies are classified according to distribution. Mononeuropathy signifies a lesion involving a single nerve, e.g., ulnar neuropathy. Mononeuropathies may result from traumatic injury to a nerve or systemic disease, such as diabetes (especially the femoral, peroneal, oculomotor, or abducens nerve).

  2. Mononeuritis multiplex indicates that several individual nerves are involved at the same time. This occurs in conjunction with systemic lupus erythematosis, rheumatoid arthritis, diabetes, and polyarteritis nodosa.

  3. Polyneuropathies are symmetrical, characteristically involving the distal aspects of the extremities with paresthesias, sensory loss, and weakness. The initial symptoms are confined to the hands and feet, the so-called stocking-glove pattern, and progress proximally. Polyneuropathies are associated with infectious, metabolic, and toxic diseases.

D. Cranial Nerves

Cranial nerve dysfunction is a frequent harbinger of an intracranial mass lesion. The basic functions of the cranial nerves are outlined in Chapter 4.

The olfactory nerve, which mediates smell, may be impaired as a result of a basilar skull fracture or an olfactory groove meningioma. Nasal congestion is the most common cause of impaired sense of smell. Uncinate fits, which may include olfactory hallucinations, do not imply actual involvement of the olfactory nerve.

Visual impulses traverse the entire sagittal extent of the brain from the retina to the occipital lobes. The optic nerves partially decussate at the optic chiasm and the axons continue back to the lateral geniculate bodies as the optic tracts. Lesions at various points along this pathway result in characteristic patterns of visual loss. These are outlined in Chapter 4. Visual loss of the entire upper or lower half of the visual field most commonly results from retinal infarction.

Extraocular motion and pupillary constriction are mediated by cranial nerves III, IV, and VI. These nerves may be affected within the brain stem by a glioma, vascular occlusion, or Wernicke's encephalopathy. They may be injured in their course through the subarachnoid space by infection, meningeal carcinomatosis, an adjacent meningioma, a chordoma, an aneurysm of the basilar or internal carotid artery, or herniation of the uncus. The pupil is characteristically dilated when the third nerve is compressed by an aneurysm or herniated uncus, but it is unaffected when the third nerve is involved in a diabetic ophthalmoplegia. An infection, a tumor, or an aneurysm involving the cavernous sinus may cause paralysis of extraocular motion. The nerves may be involved within the orbit by infection, tumor, or orbital pseudotumor.

Tic douloureux is a distinct type of lancinating trigeminal pain that has several causes. The trigeminal nerve may be compressed by an adjacent tumor in the posterior fossa, parasellar region, or cavernous sinus. The nerve may also be affected by herpes zoster and connective tissue disorders.

Facial nerve paralysis is frequently idiopathic (Bell's palsy). The Ramsay Hunt syndrome (caused by herpes zoster of the facial nerve) presents as ear and throat pain and facial weakness. Hemifacial spasm, a periodic twitching and/or tonic contraction of the facial muscles on one side, is amenable to treatment by microvascular decompression of the seventh nerve at its exit from the pons.

The eighth cranial nerve is the cranial nerve most frequently involved by a schwannoma. Several other disorders of the eighth nerve may result in vertigo, tinnitus, and/or deafness.

Disorders of the ninth, tenth, and eleventh cranial nerves may arise from infection or trauma involving the jugular foramen or carotid sheath. Meningiomas, epidermoids, and schwannomas affect these nerves within the cranial cavity, and glomus tumors affect the nerves within the jugular foramen. Glossopharyngeal neuralgia is an intermittent sharp pain in the throat triggered by stimulation of the tonsillar fossa, which can be relieved by intracranial sectioning of the glossopharyngeal nerve and part of the vagus nerve.

The hypoglossal nerve may be damaged by an inflammation of the basal meninges or the carotid sheath along with the ninth, tenth, and eleventh cranial nerves. A hypoglossal palsy may result from an atherosclerotic aneurysm of the vertebral artery or Paget's disease.

REFERENCES

Das Gupta TK: Tumors of the peripheral nerves. Clin Neurosurg 25:574-590, 1978.

Dunsker SB: Cervical Spondylosis. New York, Raven Press, 1981.

Haymaker W, Woodhall B: Peripheral Nerve Injuries: Principles of Diagnosis, ed 2. Philadelphia, WB Saunders, 1953.

Kopell HP, Thompson WAL: Peripheral Entrapment Neuropathies. Huntington, NY, Robert E. Krieger, 1976.

Murphey F: Experience with lumbar disc surgery. Clin Neurosurg 20:1-8, 1973.

Murphey F, Simmons JCH, Brunson B: Ruptured cervical discs 1939 to 1972. Clin Neurosurg 20:9-17, 1973.

Chapter 13

Infection

Infections appear on the neurosurgical service de novo or as a complication of surgical therapy.

A. Brain Abscess

   1. Source of Abscess

      a. Parameningeal. Frontal sinusitis may spread into the frontal lobe; mastoiditis may extend into the cerebellum or the posterior temporal lobe.

      b. Contamination via penetrating cranial trauma or operation. Abscesses frequently occur around retained bone fragments or foreign bodies.

      c. Hematogenous spread from pneumonia, endocarditis, etc. Patients with right to left intracardiac shunts are especially susceptible.

   2. Clinical Signs

      a. Mass effect, with headache, nausea, lethargy, and papilledema. A focal neurological deficit may be present, indicative of the area of the brain involved.

      b. Seizures.

      c. Meningeal irritation with nuchal rigidity and photophobia, if meningitis is also present.

      d. Although the primary source (e.g., sinusitis) may cause systemic symptoms and signs of infection, the brain abscess usually does not.

   3. Diagnosis

      a. Mild leukocytosis, elevated erythrocyte sedimentation rate. These may be normal.

      b. X-ray films of the skull may demonstrate paranasal sinusitis.

    c. A lumbar puncture (LP) will not make the diagnosis of a brain abscess. More importantly, an LP may lead to brain herniation if a brain abscess is present. Therefore, the safest approach is to obtain a CT brain scan before deciding to do a lumbar puncture in a patient who might have a brain abscess.

    d. CT scan: The typical appearance of a brain abscess is a contrast-enhanced rim around a center of low attenuation and a variable amount of surrounding cerebral edema.

4. Microbiology: With otitis: Streptococcus, Haemophilus influenzae, gram-negative anaerobes. With sinusitis: Streptococcus, Staphylococcus. With a penetrating wound: Staphylococcus. With hematogenous spread: various organisms (Nocardia has a propensity to seed the brain).

5. Treatment: The purpose of treatment is to eradicate the infection and eliminate the mass effect.

    a. Begin appropriate antibiotic coverage. During the stage of acute cerebritis, prior to abscess formation, surgical treatment is seldom indicated. Pending cultures (aerobic, anaerobic, and fungal), begin treatment with penicillin (>20 million units per day) or nafcillin (12 g per day), chloramphenicol (3-4 g per day), and occasionally metronidazole. Continue antibiotic treatment for 4-6 weeks. Antibiotics alone have been used successfully to eradicate early cerebral abscesses in high-risk patients.

    b. Corticosteroids reduce cerebral edema but also inhibit the formation of the abscess capsule.

    c. Surgical therapy consists of one of the following:

        i. Excision in toto without violating the abscess wall. This procedure results in a cure of the disease but if the abscess is removed from functionally important areas of the brain, the neurological deficit may be increased.

       ii. Drainage of the abscess without resection of the abscess wall. This treatment has a significant rate of recurrence.

     iii. Multiple aspirations through a trephination. This method allows a bacteriological diagnosis to be made, but satellite abscesses and loculated cavities within the abscess may not be drained.

    d. Treatment of the primary bacterial source.

6. Results: Prior to CT scanning, the mortality rate from brain abscess was 15-40%. Because the diagnosis has been simplified by CT scanning and the possibility of recurrence can be monitored with serial CT scans, the mortality rate has been diminished. Focal neurological deficits may persist, and 30-70% of patients will have postoperative seizures, which have a mean onset of 3.3 years following treatment.

B. Subdural Empyema

Subdural empyema frequently evolves from frontal sinusitis or mastoiditis but may result from a local scalp infection concomitant with osteomyelitis, infection of a pre-existing subdural hematoma, hematogenous spread of infection, or meningitis.

1. Clinical Symptoms

    a. Early symptoms from sinusitis: focal pain and swelling, fever.

    b. Later symptoms from the subdural infection: generalized headache, drowsiness, meningismus, focal seizures, focal deficit (if the abscess is interhemispheric, lower extremity weakness or a homonymous field deficit may develop).

2. Diagnosis

    a. X-ray films of the skull may demonstrate sinusitis, mastoiditis, or osteomyelitis of the skull.

    b. The CT scan reveals an extracerebral low-density mass with an enhancing capsule.

3. Organism: Streptococcus (most common), Staphylococcus, anaerobic and gram-negative organisms.

4. Treatment: This is a neurosurgical emergency.

    a. Evacuate pus through a craniectomy, or a craniotomy. Protect the arachnoid membrane to avoid subarachnoid extension of the infection (meningitis). Drainage through multiple burr holes is usually not adequate.

    b. Initiate broad-spectrum antibiotic therapy pending anaerobic and aerobic culture results (penicillin, chloramphenicol).

    c. Eradicate primary source of infection - exenterate frontal or mastoid sinuses, remove infected bone.

5. Results: Subdural empyemas have a mortality rate of 10-20%. The mortality rate becomes higher as the patient becomes less conscious.

C. Osteomyelitis

Osteomyelitis of the skull results from paranasal sinusitis, from infection of a compound fracture or a penetrating wound, or from hematogenous spread of bacteria. Symptoms include local pain and tenderness, erythema, swelling (Pott's puffy tumor), and drainage from the infected area. A concomitant epidural abscess can result in a focal neurological deficit or seizures.

X-ray films of the skull demonstrate a "moth-eaten" appearance with irregular punched-out areas. Treatment consists of debridement of necrotic bone and concomitant administration of antibiotics.

D. Craniotomy Wound Infection

Postoperative infections may involve the scalp, bone, or subdural or subarachnoid spaces. Craniotomy infections are most common in debilitated patients, following multiple craniotomies, after long operations, or when a foreign body or drain is used. The infected wound will be indurated, tender, erythematous, and edematous. Treatment consists of antibiotics and wound debridement, which includes the removal of devascularized bone. In some cases the infected wound may be treated successfully by using an irrigation-suction apparatus for 7 days to continuously irrigate the infected area with an antibiotic solution. If this is successful, the bone flap may be left in place. If infection persists, the bone is removed. After the removal of an infected bone flap, a cranioplasty may be performed, but usually a year is allowed to elapse between the two procedures to reduce the possibility of an infection about the cranioplasty plate.

E. Meningitis

Bacterial meningitis may occur after head trauma that opens the subarachnoid space to areas containing bacteria (such as the paranasal sinuses) and may also complicate a craniotomy.

1. Clinical signs: Fever, nuchal rigidity, and cerebral dysfunction (lethargy, seizures); papilledema is rare.

2. Diagnosis: Lumbar puncture - increased number of leukocytes; diminished glucose value (<40 mg per dl or less than one-half the serum glucose level). CSF lactic acid and limulus lipate assay for gram-negative rods.

3. Bacteriology:

    a. Gram-negative rods (Klebsiella, <u>Escherichia</u> <u>coli</u>, Pseudomonas) occur in association with surgery or a persistent CSF leak through a paranasal sinus or the middle ear. Gram-negative meningitis had a 60% mortality rate prior to the institution of intraventricular antibiotic therapy.

    b. <u>Staphylococcus</u> <u>aureus</u> occurs in conjunction with open head trauma, after surgery, or with a dermal sinus tract.

    c. Pneumococcus occurs after trauma with an associated persistent CSF leak.

4. Treatment:

    a. Gram-negative rods: Chloramphenicol 4-6 g per day, i.v. (resistance may develop), or moxalactam 8-12 g per day, i.v. An aminoglycoside must be given intrathecally. Since 70% of these patients have associated intraventricular infections, a Rickham or Ommaya reservoir is frequently used to facilitate intraventricular antibiotic administration. Doses: tobramycin or gentamicin 5 mg per day; amikacin 15 mg per ml of CSF per day. Concomitant systemic therapy may be used. Cultures of CSF may not become sterile for up to 10 days.

    b. <u>Staphylococcus</u> <u>aureus</u>: Nafcillin 2-3 g, i.v., q 4 h.

    c. Pneumococcus: Penicillin G 50,000 units per kg q 4 h for adult; 70,000 units per kg q 8 h for neonate.

F. Infected Shunt

Ventriculoperitoneal shunts have a 5-10% infection rate, but the rate of infection may be reduced by employing pre- and intraoperative antibiotics. The infection may present as acute sepsis soon after shunt placement or insidiously as intermittent fever, leukocytosis, and shunt malfunction. The offending organisms and antibiotic sensitivity must be identified. Some patients can be treated effectively with a combination of intraventricular and systemic antibiotics. In the remaining patients, the infected shunt must be removed.

G. Cysticercosis

Cysticercosis, a common cause of an intracranial mass in patients from Mexico, develops from an infection with the larval stage of the pork tapeworm. Cysticerci give rise to multiple vesicles in the ventricles and subarachnoid space which can act as an intracranial mass or obstruct the flow of CSF.

H. Toxoplasmosis

Toxoplasmosis of the central nervous system is a congenital infection which presents with convulsions, hydrocephalus or microcephaly, intracerebral calcifications, microphthalmia, chorioretinitis, and multiple extraneural manifestations.

I. Viral Infections

1. Herpes simplex encephalitis, which most frequently involves the inferior frontal and medial temporal lobes, presents with changes in mentation, memory loss, meningismus, or olfactory seizures. As the disease evolves, seizures and coma appear. Once the diagnosis is confirmed by biopsy, 15 mg per kg of adenosine arabinoside is given per day (via a 12-hour intravenous infusion) for 10 days.

2. Progressive multifocal leukoencephalopathy presents with multifocal neurological deficits and dementia. It occurs in association with malignancies and lymphoproliferative diseases.

3. Jakob-Creutzfeldt's disease is manifested by rapidly progressive dementia, myoclonus, spastic weakness of the extremities, and ataxia. A slow virus is thought to be the infectious agent responsible for the disease.

J. Reye's Syndrome

Reye's syndrome is a rapidly progressive encephalopathy and hepatic decompensation occurring in childhood. Following a prodromal viral infection, patients develop altered mentation, delirium, and coma. Treatment aimed at monitoring and controlling elevated intracranial pressure, treating hypoglycemia, and correcting coagulopathies has lowered the mortality rate associated with this condition.

K. Mycotic Aneurysms

Mycotic aneurysms, a consequence of septic emboli, most frequently involve the distal branches of the middle cerebral artery. Rupture of a mycotic aneurysm usually causes an intracerebral hematoma. Treatment consists of antibiotic therapy and, when possible, surgical obliteration of the aneurysm. Bacterial endocarditis, a frequent source of septic emboli, may also be responsible for embolic stroke, cerebral abscesses, or meningitis.

L. Spinal Infections

1. Spinal epidural empyema may result from the hematogenous
    spread of infection or as a complication of spinal surgery or
    lumbar puncture. Staphylococcus aureus is the most frequent
    infecting agent.

    a. Clinical presentation: The patient presents with back
        pain and perhaps concomitant radicular pain. The spine
        is tender to percussion over the lesion. As the
        infection progresses, signs of spinal cord or cauda
        equina compression appear.

    b. Laboratory studies: Fever and leukocytosis are absent
        in chronic infections and mild in acute infections.
        Spine roentgenograms may demonstrate osteomyelitis.
        Examination of the spinal fluid reveals signs of a
        parameningeal focus, i.e., elevated protein content,
        relatively mild leukocytosis, and a normal level of
        glucose. A myelogram is performed which may demonstrate
        partial or total epidural obstruction.

    c. Treatment: Surgical decompression, antibiotics, diag-
        nosis and treatment of the source of the infection.
        Rule out diabetes mellitus.

2. Spinal subdural empyema is a rare condition with a similar
    presentation as a spinal epidural abscess. Pain on spinal
    percussion is absent. Myelography demonstrates multiple
    filling defects indicating multiple foci of infection.

3. Intramedullary spinal cord infection is a rare condition
    resulting from direct contamination, infection of a dermal
    sinus, or hematogenous spread. Spinal cord dysfunction
    progresses with little pain, fever, or leukocytosis.

4. Disc space infection typically occurs in children or follow-
    ing surgical discectomy. Spontaneous vertebral osteomyelitis
    usually begins at the vertebral end plate. Staphylococcus is
    the most frequent infecting agent.

    a. Clinical signs:

        i. Severe back pain - frequently associated with
            radicular pain.

        ii. Paravertebral muscle spasms.

        iii. Local tenderness.

b. Diagnosis:

    i. An elevated erythrocyte sedimentation rate.

    ii. Leukocytosis may be present.

    iii. Radiographic changes.

        a) Narrowing of the disc space.

        b) Sclerosis of the subchondral bone.

        c) Irregularity of the adjacent vertebral end plates.

    iv. Positive blood cultures.

    v. Needle biopsy of the disc space may yield a histological and bacteriological diagnosis.

c. Treatment:

    i. Bed rest is the key to early therapy.

    ii. Immobilization in a spica or body jacket.

    iii. Antibiotics, intravenously at first and then by mouth.

    iv. Surgical decompression is only indicated if there is a concomitant paravertebral or epidural abscess.

5. Pott's disease, tuberculous osteomyelitis of the spine, most frequently involves the thoracic spine. X-ray films reveal collapse of adjacent vertebral bodies and obscuration of the disc margins. Epidural or paravertebral abscesses are common.

M. Antibiotics

The penicillins and chloramphenicol are the most frequently employed antibiotics used to treat CNS infection. Metronidazole, because of its impressive potency in combating anaerobic organisms, is used to treat otogenic brain abscesses. The aminoglycosides are used to treat infections caused by gram-negative rods. Lincomycin, erythromycin, tetracycline, and the first and second generation cephalosporins are rarely used in the therapy of CNS infections (see Table 13.1).

Table 13.1.
Antibiotics for the Treatment for Meningitis

Drug	Penetrates into CSF	Dose
Penicillin G	Fair[*]	20-24 million units/d i.v. adult (q 4 h) 0.15-0.4 million units/d i.v. child (q 4 h)
Nafcillin	Fair[†]	12 g/d i.v. (q 4 h) 75 mg/d intrathecal
Methicillin	Fair[†]	16-24 g/d i.v. 25-100 mg/d intrathecal
Ampicillin	Fair[†]	12 g/d i.v. adult (q 4 h) 200-400 mg/kg/d i.v. child (q 4 h) 50 mg/d intrathecal
Carbenicillin	Fair[†]	30 g/d i.v. adult (q 4 h) 300-500 mg/kg/d i.v. child (q 4 h) (rarely used) 75 mg intraventricular (q 8 h)
Chloramphenicol	Good	3-4 g/d i.v. adult (q 6 h) 50-100 mg/kg/d i.v. child (q 6 h)
Cephalothin	Poor	4-12 g/d i.v. (q 6 h) 25-100 mg/d intrathecal
Cephaloridine	Poor	2-4 g/d i.v. (q 6 h) 12.5-50 mg intrathecal qod
Tetracycline	Fair[†]	50 mg/kg/d i.v. (q 6 h)
Lincomycin	Poor	(Rarely used) 3-8 g/d i.v. adult (q 6 h) 10-20 mg/kg/d i.v. child (q 8 h) 1-2 mg/d intrathecal
Erythromycin	Poor	2 g/d p.o. (q 6 h) (Rarely used) 1-10 mg/d intrathecal

Table 13.1. (cont'd)

Drug	Penetrates into CSF	Dose
Vancomycin	Fair[†]	40-50 mg/kg/d i.v. (q 6 h) 5-10 mg/d intrathecal (q 12-24 h)
Polymixin B	Poor	2.5 mg/kg/d i.v. (q 8 h) 0.03 mg/kg/d intrathecal
Gentamicin	Poor	3-5 mg/kg/d i.v. adult (q 8 h) 7.5 mg/kg/d i.v. child (q 8 h) 1 mg/kg/d intrathecal child 5-10 mg/kg/d intrathecal (q 12-24 h)
Tobramycin	Poor	3-5 mg/kg/d i.v. adult (q 8 h) 7.5 mg/kg/d i.v. child 5-10 mg/d intrathecal (q 12-24 h)
Amikacin	Poor	15 mg/kg/d i.v. (q 8 h) 15 mg/d intrathecal
Trimethaprim/ Sulfamethoxazole	Good	40 ml/d i.v. (q 12 h)
Metronidazole	Good	1200-1800 mg/d i.v. (q 8 h)
Rifampin	Good	600 mg/d p.o. adult (q 12 h) 10 mg/kg/d p.o. child (q 12 h) 0.5-1 mg/d intrathecal
Isoniazid	Good	300 mg/d i.m. or p.o. adult (q day) 15 mg/kg/d i.m. or i.v. child (q day)
Amphotericin	Poor	0.3-1.0 mg/kg/d i.v. 0.1-0.3 mg three times per week
Para Aminosalicylic Acid	Poor	6 g/d adult (q 12 h) 150 mg/kg/d child (q 24 h)
5-Fluorocytosine	Poor	150 mg/kg/d (q 6 h)

Table 13.1. (cont'd)

Drug	Penetrates into CSF	Dose
Miconazole	Poor	1.8-3.6 g/d i.v. (q 8 h) 20 mg/d intrathecal
Ketoconazole	Poor	0.4-0.8 mg/kg p.o.
Moxalactam	Good	2-12 g/d i.v. adult (q 8 h) 150-200 mg/kg child (q 8 h)
Cefotaxime	Fair	4-12 g/d i.v. (q 8 h)
Sulfazoxole	Good	g/d i.v. (q 6 h)

*Poor entrance into CSF compensated for by large blood concentration.

†Crosses the blood-brain barrier poorly in the absence of infection.

REFERENCES

Bannister G, William B, Smith S: Treatment of subdural empyema. J Neurosurg 55:82-88, 1981.

Bell WE: Treatment of bacterial infections of the central nervous system. Ann Neurol 9:313-327, 1981.

Bell WE: Treatment of fungal infections of the central nervous system. Ann Neurol 9:417-422, 1981.

Buckwold FJ, Hand R, Hansebout RR: Hospital-acquired bacterial meningitis in neurosurgical patients. J Neurosurg 46:494-500, 1977.

Everett ED, Strausbaugh LJ: Antimicrobial agents and the central nervous system. Neurosurgery 6:691-714, 1980.

Samson DS, Clark K: A current review of brain abscess. Am J Med 54:201-210, 1973.

Wilson N: Infections of the Nervous System. Philadelphia, FA Davis, 1979.

Chapter 14

Seizures

Seizures are commonly encountered in the neurosurgeon's practice in association with cerebral contusion, stroke, intracranial hematoma, and brain tumor. Focal seizures are especially prone to occur during the immediate postoperative period. Although some neurosurgeons give patients prophylactic anticonvulsants prior to a craniotomy, the efficacy of this regimen in preventing postoperative seizures has not been substantiated.

Seizures are classified as generalized or partial (focal). All forms of seizures begin in a focal area of abnormally discharging cells, but in primary generalized seizures, there are no clues as to the location of the abnormal locus.

A. Partial Seizures

1. Focal epilepsy is always due to a focal cortical lesion. Focal seizures are classified as:

    a. Elementary (without loss of consciousness).

    b. Complex (associated with an altered consciousness).

    c. Focal seizures with secondary generalization.

2. The location of the cortical seizure focus will determine the initial manifestations of the seizure. Because the patient may not remember the first manifestations of the seizure, a history from someone who observed the seizure will be helpful. Signs which localize the focal lesion are:

    a. Anterior frontal lobe: turning of head and eyes to the opposite side.

    b. Motor cortex: tonic-clonic movements in the opposite limbs/trunk/face.

    c. Sensory cortex: focal paresthesias in the opposite limbs/trunk/face.

    d. Occipital lobe: scintillations or transient visual field deficits in the contralateral half of each visual

153

field (well formed images are produced by temporal lobe seizures).

   e. Temporal: auditory, olfactory, vertiginous, or visceral hallucinations.

3. Complex partial seizures frequently begin with a focal temporal lobe aura, and then the patient develops a change in consciousness associated with a complex hallucination or perceptual abnormality. These include:

   a. Déjà vu: the incorrect illusion that a new situation is the repetition of a previous situation.

   b. Automatisms: the performance of nonreflex movements without conscious volition.

   c. Changes in mood: fear, depression, anxiety.

   d. Formed hallucinations: objects may appear small and distant or large.

4. Temporary postictal neurological deficits may help localize the origin of the seizures, e.g., postictal paralysis (Todd's paralysis).

B. Generalized Seizures

1. Tonic-clonic seizures may have a prodromal mood change lasting hours to days. The patient then loses consciousness, becomes rigid, and proceeds to have synchronous spasms of the face, trunk, and limbs. These attacks are followed by a postictal period of confusion and drowsiness. These can occur following withdrawal from alcohol or barbiturates or in association with metabolic abnormalities (i.e., uremia, hypoglycemia).

2. Petit mal seizures are brief lapses in consciousness lasting only a few seconds during which the patient does not speak and does not understand verbal commands. These are seen in childhood and have a characteristic EEG abnormality of a 3 per second spike and wave pattern.

3. Akinetic seizures are generalized seizures associated with loss of postural tone and falling.

C. Evaluation

1. In the postoperative patient, a seizure may be the harbinger of an evolving problem, such as an electrolyte imbalance, abnormal blood pH, infection, intraparenchymal hematoma, or subdural hematoma.

2. In the unoperated adult patient, alcohol or barbiturate withdrawal, neoplasm, encephalitis, metabolic abnormalities (e.g., uremia, hyponatremia), stroke, degenerative disease, and rarely subarachnoid hemorrhage should be considered.

3. Laboratory tests include:

   a. EEG for localization.

   b. Metabolic screen.

   c. Serum anticonvulsant levels, when indicated.

   d. CT scan of the brain.

   e. Lumbar puncture.

D. Treatment

1. Medical therapy is initiated by starting one drug at a time. The initial drug is increased until the seizures have abated or a maximum therapeutic serum level of the drug is reached prior to initiating a second medication.

   a. Generalized and focal seizures are treated with phenytoin, phenobarbital, or carbamazepine.

   b. Minor seizures have been included in the discussion for completeness although they are seldom a neurosurgical problem. These attacks should be treated with ethosuximide, clonazepam, or valproic acid.

   c. The withdrawal of drugs after a seizure-free period always carries the risk of recurrent seizures. Some physicians will slowly withdraw anticonvulsants if the patient remains seizure free for 2 years and the EEG demonstrates no epileptiform activity.

2. Surgical therapy is reserved for patients who have a well localized focus of seizure activity which is refractory to medical management. Most frequently this involves a temporal lobectomy for seizures emanating from the mesial temporal lobe or hemispherectomy in children with childhood hemiplegia and intractable seizures. This surgery is only performed in specially equipped units.

Table 14.1.
Anticonvulsant Drugs

Drug	Daily Dose	Therapeutic Level	Common Side Effects
Phenytoin	300-500 mg	10-20 µg/ml	Nystagmus, ataxia, dermatitis, osteomalacia, gingival hyperplasia, systemic lupus erythematosus, blood dyscrasia, hirsutism
Phenobarbital	45-180 mg	15-30 µg/ml	Ataxia, sedation, irritability, hyperactivity, rash
Primidone	250-1500 mg	5-12 µg/ml	Ataxia, lethargy, rash, leukopenia
Ethosuximide	250-1500 mg	40-120 µg/ml	Nausea, dizziness, systemic lupus erythematosus, rash, blood dyscrasia
Carbamazepine	600-1200 mg	4-8 µg/ml	Diplopia, dizziness, drowsiness, anorexia, blood dyscrasia
Valproic acid	1000-3000 mg	50-100 µg/ml	Nausea, vomiting, hepatic toxicity
Clonazepam	0.6-1.2 mg	0.025-0.075 µg/ml	Irritability, aggressiveness, ataxia, blood dyscrasias

E.   Status Epilepticus

Status epilepticus occurs when the patient does not recover
consciousness between seizures. The patient may have continuous
tonic-clonic movement or no movement at all. The only signs of
status epilepticus may be a tonic deviation of the eyes or a

slight twitching of a finger. These small clues should be looked
for in patients with unexplained coma.

Treatment of status epilepticus:

1. Establish an adequate airway and maintain oxygenation.
    Monitor electrocardiogram and blood pressure.

2. Recurrent seizures are particularly difficult to suppress in
    the face of a persistent electrolyte abnormality. Alkalosis
    and hypomagnesemia are common abnormalities in alcoholics
    with persistent seizures. Draw blood for determination of
    arterial pH, PO_2, PCO_2, and venous anticonvulsant levels,
    glucose, electrolytes, and blood urea nitrogen.

3. Anticonvulsants are given one at a time. Most of these drugs
    are respiratory depressants. Diazepam, phenytoin, or
    phenobarbital should be tried first. If they are not
    successful, paraldehyde, lidocaine, or sodium amytal may be
    employed.

4. If all anticonvulsant therapy fails, general anesthesia can
    be used to stop the seizures.

5. Continuous focal seizures are not a medical emergency. They
    are frequently seen in the postoperative period because of
    local cortical irritation. They also occur as a result of
    a stroke, a local cerebral infection, or a hematoma.

Table 14.2
Drugs Used in the Treatment of Status Epilepticus

Drug	Dose	Instructions	Side Effects
Phenytoin	50 mg/min	Dilute in normal saline; slow infusion; EKG monitor essential for arrhythmias; loading dose 1 g	Prolonged PR interval and QRS wave; vascular collapse
Phenobarbital	25 mg/min	Infuse as 120 mg bolus q 15 min until 600 mg	Hypotension and respiratory depression

Table 14.2 (cont'd)

Drug	Dose	Instructions	Side Effects
Diazepam	5-10 mg	Infuse no faster than 2 mg/min; repeat q 10 min until maximum of 30 mg	Respiratory depression
Paraldehyde	Infusion initiated to control seizures	5 ml paraldehyde in 500 ml 5% dextrose in water (4% solution)	Respiratory depression; infiltration of i.v. can lead to tissue necrosis
Sodium amytal	Infusion initiated to control seizures	200-1000 mg i.v.	Respiratory depression
Lidocaine	50-100 mg i.v. push	If lidocaine is effective, institute a continuous intravenous infusion of 1-2 mg/min	Seizures, arrhythmias

REFERENCES

Anneggers JF, Grabow JD, Groover RV, et al: Seizures after head trauma: a population study. Neurology 30:683-689, 1980.

Delgado-Escueta AV, Wasterlain C, Treiman DM, et al: Current concepts in neurology: management of status epilepticus. N Engl J Med 306:1337-1340, 1982.

Millichap JG: Drug treatment of convulsive disorders. N Engl J Med 286:464-469, 1972.

Sutherland JM, Eadie MJ: The Epilepsies: Modern Diagnosis and Treatment. Edinburgh, Churchill Livingstone, 1980.

Chapter 15

Pain

The physician initially confronts pain as the signal of some underlying disease. Treatment is aimed at eradicating the underlying disorder responsible for the pain. Occasionally an underlying problem cannot be eradicated or even identified. In these cases, pain becomes the patient's primary problem.

A. Anatomy (Fig. 15.1)

In the past 10 years significant strides have been made in elucidating the anatomical substrates of pain. Peripheral receptors responsible for pain (nociceptors) are activated by mechanical or chemical stimuli. Agents present at the site of inflammation--such as bradykinin, histamine, prostaglandins, and serotonin--are capable of stimulating chemosensitive nociceptors. Prostaglandins sensitize the receptors, lowering the receptors' threshold to other stimuli.

Afferent nerves mediating painful stimuli are of a small diameter (A-delta and C). These nerves make their first synaptic connection in the dorsal horn of the spinal cord. Cells in the dorsal horn, which are excited by small-diameter fibers, are inhibited by larger diameter fibers (A-alpha and beta) which mediate nonpainful signals (the gate theory of pain). Single neurons conveying painful impulses from the dorsal horn to the ventral posterolateral thalamus are grouped in the ventrolateral part of the spinal cord (spinothalamic tract). These fibers are responsible for sharp, well localized pain. Other multisynaptic pathways convey painful impulses to the brain stem, thalamus, and limbic system. These pathways are responsible for dull, burning, poorly localized pain and affective components of pain.

Descending pathways from the brain stem (periaqueductal gray matter) can modulate painful impulses in the dorsal horn. This supressive system employs endorphin, serotonin, and norepinephrine receptors.

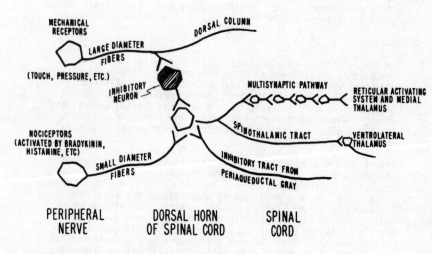

PERIPHERAL   DORSAL HORN   SPINAL
  NERVE   OF SPINAL CORD   CORD

Figure 15.1. Pain pathways.

B. Drug Therapy

    1. Drugs aimed at suppressing pain can act at various places
        along the pain pathway.
        a. Chemosensitive nociceptors: steroids, nonsteroid anti-
            inflammatory agents (acetylsalicylate, zomepirac, etc.).

        b. Afferent fibers: injection of local anesthetics.

        c. Descending central pain modulating circuits: narcotics,
            antidepressants.

2. Psychotropic and antidepressant drugs are used for the
    affective component of the pain. These drugs do not
    eliminate the pain but reduce the amount of suffering
    associated with the pain. These drugs may also have an
    effect on the pain pathways.

    a. Chlorpromazine and haloperidol are used as an adjuvant
        in treating chronically painful injuries.

    b. Amitriptyline, sometimes in conjunction with
        fluphenazine, is used in chronic pain syndromes.
        Amitriptyline has proved to be especially effective in
        the treatment of painful diabetic neuropathy.

3. Postoperative pain following a cranial operation is usually
    mild. The patient should not receive strong narcotics which
    will alter cognitive functions. Following a spinal
    operation, the patient may require strong narcotics (morphine
    sulfate 10-12 mg i.m. q 3-4 h) for adequate pain relief.

4. Patients suffering with chronic pain of a nonmalignant
    origin should be treated with nonaddicting, non-narcotic
    analgesics and psychotropic medications.

5. When the underlying cause of cancer pain cannot be corrected,
    analgesics are employed. Mild pain is treated with non-
    narcotic analgesics. Severe pain can be mitigated by small
    doses of methadone (5-20 mg p.o.) given every 6 hours. This
    regular regimen anticipates the patient's pain and appears to
    be more effective than the administration of narcotics only
    when the pain becomes intolerable. The regular dose of
    methadone may be supplemented by Hospice mix (morphine,
    phenothiazine, and alcohol) or Brompton's mixture (morphine,
    cocaine, alcohol, and chloroform water).

C. Psychiatric Therapy

    Depression frequently accentuates chronic pain. Psychological
    intervention may be an important component of pain management.
    This consists of:

    1. Psychotropic drugs.

    2. Behavior modification.

    3. Biofeedback and hypnosis.

D. Electrical Stimulation

    Electrical stimulation of peripheral nerves or the dorsal columns
    of the spinal cord is used in the treatment of chronic pain.
    Theoretically this electrically stimulates large sensory fibers

which in turn inhibit the passage of painful stimuli beyond the spinal level (see "Anatomy"). Although only one-third of pain patients get satisfactory relief of pain with stimulation alone, another third receive some relief which aids in their overall management.

E. Ablative Surgery

Ablative surgery has proven beneficial in treating certain types of pain. Successful relief of pain is most often obtained when the limitations of the particular procedure are known and honored.

1. Alcohol injection, avulsion, or section of a branch of the trigeminal nerve is sometimes carried out in the treatment of trigeminal neuralgia. Similar procedures may be performed on peripheral nerves in the treatment of a painful neuroma. The relief obtained by these techniques is usually temporary.

2. Dorsal rhizotomies, the interruption of the dorsal (sensory) nerve roots within the spinal canal, are accomplished by surgically dividing the roots through a laminectomy. Multiple rhizotomies may be performed by bathing the nerve roots with intrathecal phenol (suspended in oil) or alcohol administered through a lumbar puncture. A similar effect may be obtained by cauterizing the nerve root within the neural foramen. The cautery needle may be guided into the neural foramen with the help of fluoroscopy (percutaneous rhizotomy). For dorsal rhizotomies to be effective, all of the overlapping dermatomes which supply the painful area must be blocked. This precludes the use of rhizotomies in the management of large areas of pain.

3. Retrogasserian rhizotomy, the destruction of sensory fibers of the trigeminal nerve, can also be performed by the percutaneous method. This operation is frequently successful in treating tic douloureux.

4. Sympathectomy is used to treat causalgic pain and visceral pain. Celiac ganglion blocks have been especially helpful in treating pain associated with pancreatic disease.

5. Surgically produced dorsal root entry zone lesions in the spinal cord are especially helpful in treating phantom limb pain or the pain associated with discrete spinal cord lesions.

6. Cordotomy, the surgical interruption of the spinothalamic tract, results in hemianalgesia below the level of the operation. Although this procedure is effective in managing unilateral pain associated with metastatic cancer, its efficacy diminishes with time; within 1 year after the

procedure, up to 20% of patients develop painful dysesthesias in the anesthetic area. This procedure is usually
performed percutaneously at the C1-2 level with the patient
awake. Risks involved in bilateral high cervical cordotomy
include sleep-induced apnea (Ondine's curse) and bladder,
bowel, and sexual dysfunction. Commissural myelotomy is a
longitudinal sectioning of the spinal cord in the sagittal
plane to disrupt the crossing fibers to the spinothalamic
tract.

7. Mesencephalotomy, which reduces the number of functioning
   ascending fibers in the newer specific and older nonspecific
   pain pathways, is especially effective for pains of the neck,
   head, and upper chest caused by cancer.

8. Hypophysectomy is effective in relieving bone pain associated
   with disseminated carcinoma of the breast and prostate gland.
   The pituitary gland can be removed by a trans-sphenoidal
   approach. Pain relief may also be obtained by injecting the
   pituitary with absolute alcohol.

9. Certain intracranial surgical lesions have proven to be of
   value in treating refractory pain disorders. These
   procedures can be performed stereotactically under local
   anesthesia.

   a. Surgical targets within the thalamus are the paracentral
      and lateral central nuclei which are involved in the
      primitive and poorly localized perceptions of pain.

   b. Cingulotomy involves the creation of bilateral frontal
      lesions in the medial aspects of the cerebral
      hemispheres, which modify the patient's response to the
      pain.

   After each of these central lesions, the patient still feels
   the painful sensation but no longer has the concomitant
   suffering.

E. Painful Syndromes

1. Tic douloureux presents as sharp, lightning-like paroxysms of
   pain usually confined to one or both of the two lower divi-
   sions of the trigeminal nerve. The painful events may be
   precipitated by touching a sensitive area of the face,
   chewing, or talking. Tic douloureux is usually idiopathic
   but may be associated with multiple sclerosis or a mass
   lesion in the middle or posterior fossa. Initial treatment
   consists of carbamazepine 400-1,200 mg per day or phenytoin
   100 mg t.i.d. Several surgical procedures have been employed
   in this disorder, including microvascular decompression or
   rhizotomy in the posterior fossa, percutaneous rhizolysis,

and alcohol injection or avulsion of one of the peripheral branches of the trigeminal nerve.

2. Glossopharyngeal neuralgia presents with lancinating pain in the region of the tonsil and inner ear.

3. Raeder's paratrigeminal neuralgia is a unilateral periorbital ache associated with Horner's syndrome. When this syndrome is accompanied by other cranial nerve deficits, a parasellar mass lesion should be suspected.

4. Thalamic pain, seen most frequently in conjunction with a posterior thalamic stroke, presents as paroxysms of intense aching or burning pain frequently radiating to the entire half of the body. The patients have an elevated sensory threshold, but once the threshold is reached, the stimulus may provoke paroxysms of long-lasting pain.

5. Postherpetic neuralgia is the persistence of pain after the vesicles of herpes zoster have cleared. The pain, which most often occurs in older patients, is burning in character and follows a dermatomal distribution. The thoracic dermatomes and the ophthalmic division of the trigeminal nerve are the most frequently involved areas.

6. A neuroma is an abortive attempt of axons at the site of a nerve injury to restore nerve function. The neuroma, consisting of a tangle of sprouting axons, Schwann cells, and connective tissue, occurs at the proximal end of a lacerated nerve or a partially divided nerve trunk. The pain may occur spontaneously and is exacerbated by pressure against the neuroma.

7. Causalgia refers to severe burning pain and sympathetic dystrophy seen most commonly as a result of a partial nerve injury. The patient avoids cutaneous and emotional stimuli and seeks relief by submerging the extremity in water.

8. Phantom limb pain is intractable pain which occurs after traumatic amputation. The patient frequently senses the absent limb to be held in a contorted position. Surgical lesions placed in the dorsal root entry zone will alleviate this pain in two-thirds of patients.

REFERENCES

Black P: Management of cancer pain: an overview.   Neurosurgery
5:507-518, 1979.

Ignelzi RJ, Atkinson JH: Pain and its modulation.   Neurosurgery
6:577-590, 1980.

Jannetta PJ, Robbins LJ: Trigeminal neuropathy: new observations.
Neurosurgery 7:347-351, 1980.

Kerr FWL: The Pain Book. Englewood Cliffs, NJ, Prentice-Hall, 1981.

King RB: Principles of pain management: a short review. J Neurosurg
50:554-559, 1979.

Nashold BS, Bullitt E: Dorsal root entry zone lesions to control
central pain in paraplegics. J Neurosurg 55:414-419, 1981.

Sweet WH: Percutaneous cordotomy. In Schmidek HH, Sweet WH: Current
Techniques in Operative Neurosurgery. New York, Grune & Stratton,
1972, pp 449-468.

White JC, Sweet WH: Pain and the Neurosurgeon: A Forty-year
Experience. Springfield, Charles C Thomas, 1969.

Wilkins RH: Tic douloureux. In Tindall GT, Long DM: Contemporary
Neurosurgery. Baltimore, Williams & Wilkins, 1979.

Index

167